ALZHEIMER'S DISEASE AND DEMENTIA

WHAT EVERYONE NEEDS TO KNOW®

ALZHEIMER'S DISEASE AND DEMENTIA

WHAT EVERYONE NEEDS TO KNOW®

STEVEN R. SABAT

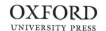

OXFORD
UNIVERSITY PRESS

OXFORD
UNIVERSITY PRESS

Oxford University Press is a department of the University of Oxford. It furthers the University's objective of excellence in research, scholarship, and education by publishing worldwide. Oxford is a registered trade mark of Oxford University Press in the UK and certain other countries.

"What Everyone Needs to Know" is a registered trademark of Oxford University Press.

Published in the United States of America by Oxford University Press 198 Madison Avenue, New York, NY 10016, United States of America.

Library of Congress Cataloging-in-Publication Data
Names: Sabat, Steven R., author.
Title: Alzheimer's disease and dementia : what everyone needs to know / Steven R. Sabat.
Description: New York, NY : Oxford University Press, [2018] | Includes bibliographical references and index.
Identifiers: LCCN 2017002631 (print) | LCCN 2017005269 (ebook) | ISBN 9780190603113 (pbk. : alk. paper) | ISBN 9780190603106 (cloth : alk. paper) | ISBN 9780190603120 (pdf) | ISBN 9780190603137 (ebook)
Subjects: LCSH: Alzheimer's disease—Patients—Care. | Alzheimer's disease—Social aspects. | Dementia—Patients—Care.
Classification: LCC RC523 .S22 2017 (print) | LCC RC523 (ebook) | DDC 616.8/311—dc23
LC record available at https://lccn.loc.gov/2017002631

Hardback printed by Bridgeport National Bindery, Inc., United States of America

To my wife, Kathy Waldman, whose love, generosity, humor, and sheer goodness of heart and soul are unforgettable blessings in my life,
and
To the memory of Dr. Bob Nussenblatt, distinguished physician, healer, and researcher, devoted husband, father and grandfather, with the love that only a brother can give.

CONTENTS

6 Types of Care and the Role of Spirituality   172

PREFACE

Directors and staff members at Alzheimer's Association chapters throughout the United States have asked how I became interested in people diagnosed with Alzheimer's disease. The answer involves decades of my life. I was 10 years old when my beloved aunt Helen died. It was my first experience of the death of a loved one. My parents, grandparents, aunt, and I lived together, and I saw her every day when I was a child. For 3 years, she struggled with the effects of brain damage that occurred initially, perhaps, due to a small stroke that caused visual dysfunction but that degenerated increasingly and she experienced intractable pain requiring heavy medication to manage. When she died at the age of 44 years, there was a hole in my heart, and I discovered the truth in C. S. Lewis's insight that "grief is the price we pay for love." In the immediate aftermath of her death, I said to myself that I needed to do something with my life to help people like her. It was November 1958.

By 1980, I had earned a Ph.D. degree in Neuropsychology and was in my sixth year on the faculty of the Psychology Department at Georgetown University, where I taught undergraduate students. During that year, I spent 1 day a week at the Johns Hopkins University Hospital Alzheimer's Disease Outpatient Clinic, administering standard neuropsychological tests to people diagnosed with dementia of different types, including the Alzheimer's type. They were participating in drug studies, and the tests were among the outcome measures used to judge the drugs' efficacy. It was my first encounter with people thus diagnosed, and the memory of those people lives with me still. What I learned from the people to whom I administered those tests and from their primary care partners led me to seek other venues wherein I could learn more from them—and I do mean from them, not merely about them. After all, these people had Alzheimer's disease (AD) and other types of dementia, and they knew what it was like from the inside and I did not. So in order to understand what AD does to people, I needed teachers who knew about it intimately, who lived with it every moment of every day. Although what I was learning from and about them during the hours of testing was valuable, it was limited for two reasons: (1) There is far more to people than their test scores, and (2) hospital clinics and taking neuropsychological tests are not representative of where we live and what we do in most of our days—unless, of course, we are medical professionals. Indeed, we spend most of our lives in the everyday social world, and so it was important that I learn from people with AD and other kinds of dementia in settings more natural, more representative of the social world, than is the hospital clinic. Those settings included people's homes and an adult day center where people go for the day for social stimulation and return home in the mid to late afternoon. What people with dementia and their care partners taught me in those venues and what I learned from colleagues who were likewise interested in understanding and helping people with dementia led ultimately to this book. Let me give you some examples to set the tone for what you will find in subsequent pages.

Example 1

It was the question-and-answer period following a presentation I gave to more than 300 family care partners, people diagnosed, and some professionals at a conference organized by the Miami Valley (Ohio) chapter of the Alzheimer's Association. A man raised his hand and asked, "Do you think it's okay for me to tell people that my wife has Alzheimer's?" I replied, "Have you asked your wife how she would feel about your doing that?" He replied, "No, but she's sitting right here." I looked at her and said, "Well, ma'am, how would you feel if your husband did that?" She replied immediately, "I wish he would. I want people to know." So I looked at her husband and said, "There's your answer, sir."

Although that answer may have been the correct one for her, it may or may not be for other people diagnosed. That is not really the point here. What is important is this: Did the man ask his wife about this before this moment? Did she know that he was thinking about it? If not, why not? If he did, and if he knew that she wanted him to tell others about her diagnosis, why did he not simply take her at her word and not ask for or need my opinion? One of the many important aspects of being a good care partner is having the lines of communication open and also being open about one's own feelings regarding the diagnosis. Many of us are unknowingly hampered by the mass media facilitated stigma about AD. The effects of stigma help neither the person diagnosed nor the care partner. Do we talk openly with the person diagnosed? Do we engage him or her in the process of coping? If we do not, why don't we and how can we learn to improve?

Example 2

The woman was a mother and grandmother who was diagnosed with probable AD approximately 3 or 4 years earlier. The final item on the tests I administered required that she write a complete sentence about whatever she wished, whatever came to mind. She asked me, "Are you a doctor?" I was wearing a badge with "Ph.D." after my name and rather than engage in a discussion about how a doctor of philosophy was a doctor but not a doctor of medicine, I said simply, "Yes." The sentence she then wrote was, "It is good to hear the doctor." I was curious about that sentence because we normally do not use that expression about a face-to-face encounter. Indeed, when the entire group of medical specialists in the clinic discussed her case, the lead physician opined that her use of the word "hear" rather than "see" was an example of a *paraphasia*—an unintended language error due to AD—and that she had meant to say, "It is good to see the doctor." It is true that AD can affect spoken and written language, so it seemed only logical that she made the kind of error that the physician alleged. It was also true that throughout the hours of testing, the woman and I had enjoyed a very warm and engaging connection.

Subsequently, I spoke with her primary care partner, her adult daughter. I learned that the woman I tested was a warm and loving mother, a recent widow, that she had been married for more than 45 years, and that the marriage had been stormy due to the fact that her husband had been verbally abusive to her throughout the marriage. Immediately, I thought of the sentence she wrote. Could it be that, having endured verbal abuse during her decades-long marriage, the woman was especially sensitive to how she was addressed by others? Given that she and I had such a warm connection during the hours of testing, perhaps she really did mean to say that it was "good to *hear* the doctor." If so, then her use of the word "hear" would not have been an example of a linguistic error due to AD but, rather, a perfectly correct statement about her experience at the time, given the context of her life history.

A series of related questions followed:

1. Might this be but one example of many instances in which seemingly aberrant behavior is not really symptomatic of AD but more properly understood as appropriate and meaningful given the diagnosed person's life and experience?

2. Might such innocent errors of interpretation help to create, in the minds of care partners, further negative expectations about the person diagnosed?

3. Might those incorrect negative expectations have an untoward effect on the care partner's interaction with the person diagnosed, thereby exacerbating the effects of the brain damage produced by the disease?

4. Might such misinterpretations result because the diagnosis is the driving force behind how those actions are interpreted? In other words, if we expect to see pathology, do we see it even where it does not exist and might that ultimately have a negative effect on the person diagnosed?

5. Are there other examples of normal, intact psychological abilities that might go unnoticed in similar ways and, if so, what might they be?

6. How might the correct recognition and support of such intact abilities improve the experience and actions of the person with AD and thereby help care partners in their efforts?

Example 3

He was approximately 68 years old and diagnosed with probable AD 4 years earlier. I was about to administer a battery of neuropsychological tests to him when he said, "Doc, ya gotta find a way to give us purpose again." Even though he had deficits in certain cognitive abilities that were serious enough for him to be diagnosed years earlier, his question itself showed that his ability to think in some very important, abstract ways was intact. Specifically, he indicated by this statement that he believed that

1. it is important to have a purpose in life, a reason to live;
2. at the present time, he was lacking in that domain;
3. he needed others to help him find purpose in his life once again; and
4. his life would be improved if he could find some purpose to live.

This is sophisticated thinking that can be found in many otherwise healthy people at various times in life; the idea of seeking and finding meaning in one's life is highly valued in this culture and important to virtually everyone. That a person diagnosed 4 years earlier with probable AD could entertain those thoughts says a great deal about what a diagnosis of AD does and does not mean. To put it in the form of a question, could it be that even though a person has serious problems with memory and other important cognitive abilities as measured by neuropsychological tests, he or she can still think in ways that are as sophisticated as they are important and that are valued in people deemed healthy? If this is the case, what does it mean in terms of how such people ought to be treated by others? How is it possible for a person to experience deficits so severe as to lead to a diagnosis of AD or other types of dementia and still be so capable in other important respects?

Example 4

The man was in his early 80s. His was the oft heard story of the immigrant who came to the United States with a few dollars to his name and who ultimately built a business that was well known throughout the metropolitan Washington, DC, area. Now, he was diagnosed with probable AD and was participating in drug studies. As well, he was volunteering at the Small Business Administration, counseling young people who were interested in starting their own businesses. It may sound odd that a person diagnosed with probable AD could be providing advice to people interested in starting their own businesses, but cases such as this are not unusual. One day, I spent several hours administering standard tests to him. In many ways, he was extremely sharp and articulate and did as well as anyone possibly could have on some of the tests. On other tests, however, he showed clear deficits that reflected his diagnosis. When the testing session ended, his wife asked me how he had done. I told her, and she became terribly upset with me because, as she put it, "How can you not see that he is just a shell of the man he used to be? How can you tell me that he did well on some tests?" She continued in that vein for a bit and then sought out other professionals to complain further.

It was clear that the man had an accurate diagnosis of probable AD. His wife was aware of the hallmarks of the diagnosis and deeply, rightfully, distressed about them and what it could mean for their lives together. Just the same, this led me to wonder: Although there was no doubt about the man's losses/weaknesses in some respects, the testing did show that he possessed certain strengths that could not be denied. Instead of reacting with relief or delight upon the news that those strengths existed, his wife seemed to be calling those test results into question, actually doubting their veracity. If his wife, who lived with him each day, was doubting the existence of some of her husband's cognitive strengths and was so intensely focused on his difficulties, how might that affect the way she treated him on a daily basis? If she saw and treated him solely as a shell of the man he used to be, might that affect the way he acted and how he felt about himself? Might he feel depressed and, if so, might the depression then be viewed as a symptom of AD instead of a logical reaction to being unacknowledged for possessing some valuable abilities in the areas of thinking and understanding and interacting with others? Each of us wants to be appreciated for our good qualities and not seen solely in terms of our faults, so how would people with AD feel if they were not valued for their positive attributes? Would they feel more despondent? Or does having a diagnosis of AD mean that the person would be completely oblivious to being defined and treated solely in terms of cognitive defects and not being appreciated for his or her positive, valued qualities?

How can we learn to recognize other remaining healthy abilities, and even strengths, in people diagnosed with AD and other types of dementia without denying the reality of the deficits? What can be done to support those strengths and to work with the deficits so as to facilitate the strengths without denying the existence of the deficits? What does dementia actually mean, and what are the different types? What happens in the brain that leads to being diagnosed? What does being diagnosed mean to people? How can people thus diagnosed be affected for better and for worse in the everyday social world? What might all this mean regarding assisted living care and nursing home care for people diagnosed? These questions and many related matters are addressed in this book.

The Overall Approach of the Book

This book is part of a series of books subtitled "What Everyone Needs to Know," published by Oxford University Press. This does not mean *"Everything* that Everyone Needs to Know" because addressing that subject would require far more than one relatively small book. So in this book, out of a vast array of possible topics, I discuss a number of things about AD and other dementias that I believe everyone needs to know. I have decided on the topics based on my interactions with people diagnosed with dementia and their care partners during the past 36 years and my experience speaking to and with audiences of such people as well as professionals in the United States and in Canada, Europe, Australia, and New Zealand.

In this book, I take a *biopsychosocial* approach. This means that we will explore the biological, psychological, and social aspects of AD and some other kinds of dementia. In the biological domain, for example, what are the typical signs and symptoms involved? What areas of the brain are damaged? What happens to brain cells and their means of communicating with one another? What are the generally observed effects of the damage and how is the diagnosis made? Are there genetic components? What drugs are prescribed, what do they do, and do they help? The typical biomedical approach to illness often ends at this point, but there is more to a person than a diagnosis and the biological problems that lead to that diagnosis and treatment.

For example, there is the person who is feeling the effects of brain injury, experiencing the loss of particular abilities and/ or the diminution of others. What do these losses mean to the person and how does he or she react to them? Do many people react alike or may people react differently to the losses of certain abilities? If people react differently, why is that the case? How do people cope with those losses? These are very important questions, and that is why we explore AD and other dementias from a *psychological* point of view (the "psycho" part of the biopsychosocial approach) so that we can appreciate the subjective experience of the people diagnosed. After all, if we do not understand how the person diagnosed feels, what the world looks like, and what matters most to him or her, how can we possibly be helpful to the greatest extent? And if we do not help that person as much as possible in nonpharmacological ways, will that have an undesirable effect on those of us who are care partners as well and what emotional and economic costs may well ensue as a result? Conversely, if we do understand as well as possible the subjective experience of the person diagnosed, can that be helpful to care partners as well as to the person diagnosed? Most of us want to be understood, sympathized with, and even empathized with, and we value greatly the people who share those connections with us. Should we assume that people diagnosed with AD or other kinds of dementia feel any differently?

Thus far, we have the biological aspect and the psychological aspects outlined, but where does the *social* aspect come into play? Well, we live in a social world wherein we interact with people much of the time, enjoying relationships of different kinds, some close, others more of the acquaintance variety. Social interactions are extremely important parts of our lives. One example of how important we believe social relationships are is the fact that one of the harshest punishments we have devised for people in prison is solitary confinement—wherein a person is unable to interact socially with anyone. In the interactions we have with others, we jointly create the various relationships we have with them. These relationships form the rich and valuable social fabric of our lives. So what happens to our social relationships if we are diagnosed with AD or some other type of dementia? Often, people diagnosed experience a loss of many social relationships and thereby are unable to continue to express themselves in the ways that those relationships allowed. What would it be like to be seen mostly, if not completely, as an "Alzheimer's patient" or a "dementia patient"? What does seeing a person in that way mean in terms of how the person is treated by others? What effect might that have on one's social connections with others and also on one's inner psychological experience? How might it feel to be seen principally in terms of the one attribute (e.g., AD) that you like the least about yourself? What would you do if that were happening to you? Can one be a friend to someone with dementia? If so, how? If a person with dementia can enjoy friendships, what does it indicate about the nature and meaning of dementia? These and other questions are addressed in connection with the *social* part of the biopsychosocial model.

When you finish reading this book, you will understand what dementia means, what causes it to occur, and what happens in the brains of people who are diagnosed. In addition, you will be able to see the person, the human being, behind the diagnosis, behind the deficits, as someone in possession of certain cognitive and social–emotional strengths—as someone worthy of consideration, respect, patience, and love. You will, I hope, understand more about the person's condition than you did before reading this book, and you may be able, as a result, to sympathize with him or her and understand how he or she is trying to cope with the cognitive losses entailed in the diagnosis. That is, you will be able to see that the human being behind the diagnostic label is very often struggling with what the legendary neuropsychologist Alexander Luria called "the tenacity of the damned" to make life as good as it can be, to retain a semblance of self-respect and honor, and to avoid being a burden, especially on those he or she loves most dearly. Perhaps it is not hyperbolic to say that you will see that dementia does not, by itself, strip a person of his or her dignity, of his or her humanity. You will learn how to identify and facilitate the diagnosed person's remaining strengths, how to communicate effectively even though the person diagnosed may have difficulty creating syntactically correct sentences, by finding the "gist" of what the person is trying to say and how to confirm the accuracy of what you believe that "gist" to be. You will learn how to set some logical limits on what you can do to make things right and how to accept what needs to be accepted in living with persons with dementia. One such reality is the fact that you cannot "make it all better." As well, you will learn that just because you cannot make it all better does not mean that you cannot make it better at all. And you will learn to put yourself in the position of the person diagnosed and thereby develop compassion to a degree that you may not have believed possible previously.

In the end, you might even discover that working together with persons diagnosed may actually be a means of grace for everyone, even though living with a person diagnosed with Alzheimer's or another type of dementia is hardly a simple task. It is a challenge to all of us to see the best in each other, to do the best for each other, and to cope as well as we can while listening to what Lincoln called "the better angels of our nature." I believe that the way we engage people diagnosed with AD or another type of dementia is a reflection of our own humanity and the degree to which that humanity can grow ever more deeply. The driving force behind my work with people diagnosed has been my belief in the strength of the human spirit in the face of consequential brain injury and in the value of humane treatment coupled with clear understanding of what dementia means and does not mean. As a result, I have been able to make good moments with such people. Good moments can add up to a good hour and perhaps a good day for people diagnosed and those deemed healthy as well. People diagnosed with AD and other dementias and their care partners have, in their interactions with me, demonstrated extraordinary courage, kindness, vulnerability, and generosity and have thereby added greatly to my life. I hope that this book and their stories will add greatly to yours.

Steven R. Sabat
Washington, DC

ACKNOWLEDGMENTS

I could not have written this book without having learned a great deal from many exceptional people. Among them, most importantly, are the following, diagnosed with Alzheimer's disease or another form of dementia, who were my teachers: Dr. B, Dr. M, Gen. U, Mrs. D, Dr. C, Mrs. E, Mrs. L, Mr. R, Mrs. K, Mr. B, Fr. O'B, Mrs. A, Mr. M, Dr. J, Mrs. F, Fr. H, Mr. N, Mrs. R, Fr. D, Mr. C, Mrs. C-B, Ms. S, Ms. B, Mr. S, and their families. Their generosity and courage in the face of daunting illness exemplify the best of what it means to be human. Although I can never repay my debt to them fully, I shall continue trying by "paying it forward."

As well, there are kindred spirits who worked wholeheartedly on "the front lines," so to speak, helping those diagnosed and their care partners and who, in the process, taught me a great deal about enlightened caregiving. My deep thanks go to Jim MacRae, the late Bob Grossman, Beth Shapiro, and Tammy Duell, former directors of the Holy Cross Hospital Medical Adult Day Center in Silver Spring, Maryland, who generously allowed my Georgetown University undergraduate students and me to become part of the community at the day center for more than 30 years so that we could learn from and give to the participants and staff there. Likewise, I thank former social workers at the day center, Marji Grossman and Erin Howard, and staff members Willie Nicole, Sr. Kathy Weber,

Patty McCabe, RN, Meg McKenna, RN, Eleanor Preston, Erv Towson, Mickie Smith, Margaret Oliu, the late Linda Parker, and Beth Montgomery, from whom I learned so very much as they worked diligently to respect and support the humanity and dignity of the day center's clients.

Through their illuminating, dedicated research, Professors Sharon Arkin, Michael Bavidge, Dawn Brooker, Christine Bryden, Rik Cheston, Jiska Cohen-Mansfield, Linda Clare, Victoria Cotrell, Murna Downs, Patrick Doyle, Kate de Medeiros, Bill Fulford, Michael Gordon, Janice Graham, Rom Harré, Penny Harris, Lars-Christer Hydén, Martha Holstein, Karen Hooker, Steve Iliffe, Kathy Kahn-Dennis, John Keady, John Killick, Tom Kitwood, Pia Kontos, Leah Light, Rebecca Logsdon, Elizabeth Lokon, Jill Manthorpe, Colin McDonnell, John McLeod, Mary Mittleman, Ali Moghaddam, Darby Morhardt, Wendy Moyle, Mike Nolan, Deb O'Connor, J. P. Orange, Stephen Post, Dorothy Pringle, Svenja Sachweh, Pamela Saunders, Claire Surr, Kate Swaffer, Dot Weaks, Carol Whitlatch, Peter Whitehouse, Bob Woods, Dan Yashinsky, Steven Zarit, and Dr. Al Power have revealed multitudes about the lives and strengths of people diagnosed with Alzheimer's and other types of dementia, as well as what exceptional caregiving entails. I am grateful to, and filled with admiration for, them. I am grateful as well to Professor Darlene Howard for teaching me about implicit memory systems and Professor Jim Lamiell for illuminating the problems inherent in applying inferential statistics to individual people.

Professor Julian Hughes's fundamentally important insights regarding how people with dementia are thought of and treated and the philosophical and ethical dimensions thereof have been of inestimable value to me. His exceptionally thoughtful books and articles are gifts to all who seek to improve the lives of people with dementia and their carers. He generously provided cogent comments and helpful suggestions in reviewing this book. Lisa Snyder's keen, sensitive understanding of people diagnosed with Alzheimer's disease and of their care partners and her extraordinary ability to facilitate the expression of their strengths in support groups, in addition to her reports thereof in her book and articles, have been powerfully instructive to me. I am tremendously fortunate to have known and learned from both of them and am blessed by their friendship.

During my 40 years on the faculty at Georgetown University, my wonderful undergraduate students' open, sharp minds, fresh perspectives, and their questions concerning people with brain injuries taught me multitudes. I shall be ever grateful to them as well for their curiosity and authenticity; they give me great hope for the future.

This book came into being principally because of Lucy Randall, my editor at Oxford University Press (OUP), whose faith in me and in this project was of signal importance from the beginning. Her thoughtful, conscientious help and guidance made writing and the process of publishing the book a joy. Hannah Doyle, Editorial Assistant at OUP, has likewise been tremendously helpful with regard to many important details and in her open, genuine interaction with me. Dan Hays provided wonderfully careful copyediting. His suggestions reflected his very close reading of the manuscript, clearly indicating that he treated his work as an art.

Finally, if not for my late parents encouraging me strongly to seek and define my own happiness and fulfillment and the examples they set of acting humanely toward others, this book would not have been written and the story of my life may well have been entirely different. My love for and gratitude to them live on.

Professor Elizabeth "Like" Lokon, Director of the Opening Minds Through Art program (OMA) at the Scripps Gerontology Center at Miami University of Ohio gave me permission to use one of the photographs from the program on the cover of this book. I am grateful for that as well as for the profoundly important work she has done to help unlock the creativity in people diagnosed with dementia.

ALZHEIMER'S DISEASE AND DEMENTIA

WHAT EVERYONE NEEDS TO KNOW®

1

DEMENTIA

People have often asked me questions such as "Is Alzheimer's worse than dementia?" or "When will we find a cure for dementia?" So, even though this book is titled *Alzheimer's Disease and Dementia*, it would make sense first to understand what dementia itself means, given that Alzheimer's disease (AD) and other illnesses can cause something that is called dementia. During most of the 20th century, dementia was understood primarily from a biomedical point of view, meaning that people diagnosed were "patients" and physicians had a monopoly on the expertise involved in "managing" their patients, with the word "managing" being the current way of saying "providing care for" patients. Medical professionals assumed that the deficits and alterations in behavior that they and family members observed in people diagnosed with dementia were caused directly by brain damage. Therefore, it was assumed that the only treatment for this condition was biomedical, similar to the approach used by physicians in their treatment of the symptoms of other illnesses. As I discussed briefly in the Preface, however, the biomedical point of view is only one way to understand dementia. There is some truth to the idea that there are 360 different ways to see an elephant. Likewise, there are ways to understand dementia other than the biomedical approach. So let's begin with an introduction to what dementia is, what it means, and what it does not mean.

Is dementia a disease?

No it is not. It is a *syndrome* because it is a group of signs (something detected by a professional) and symptoms (something experienced by the person ailing) that are correlated. These signs and symptoms can be caused by a number of different diseases that cause brain damage, including AD, Parkinson's disease, HIV/AIDS, and vascular disease that can cause small strokes. Although AD causes the largest number of instances of dementia, approximately 60–70 percent of the cases (World Health Organization, 2015), people can be diagnosed with dementia and not have AD.

Does a diagnosis of dementia mean that the person is demented?

Definitely not. It is terribly unfortunate that many people, including medical professionals (physicians and nurses) and professionals in related fields such as neuropsychology, frequently state that they have a "demented patient" or that a person is "dementing" when referring to someone diagnosed with dementia. *Demented* means crazy, unhinged, irrational, insane, or to be without a mind, according to any number of dictionaries. Clearly, being diagnosed with a type of dementia is not synonymous with being demented.

Why is it important to make the distinction between dementia and demented?

To think of a person who has been diagnosed with dementia as demented is not only incorrect but also potentially dangerous for all concerned. It is dangerous for the person diagnosed to be thought of as demented because he or she will then be treated unwittingly *as if* he or she were insane, irrational, and the like even though he or she is not. If a person is viewed as being crazy and treated as such when he or she is not crazy at all, it could result in serious psychological and emotional harm to the person as well as to his or her loved ones. It is dangerous for the professional to think of the person diagnosed as being demented because such thinking can lead to pharmacological and nonpharmacological treatment that is potentially harmful for the person diagnosed and his or her loved ones, as well as undermining the well-meaning efforts of the medical professionals. In this sense, it could mean violating the Hippocratic Oath "to do no harm." Knowing that a diagnosis of dementia does not mean that the person is demented leads to the next question.

What is the definition of the syndrome called dementia?

According to the fifth edition of the *Diagnostic and Statistical Manual of Mental Disorders* (American Psychiatric Association, 2013), dementia is now called a major neurocognitive disorder. This means that it is caused by brain damage (neuro) that affects negatively one's ability to engage in certain kinds of thinking and action (cognitive). Specifically, dementia entails a decline from previous levels of ability in one or more of the following areas:

- Learning
- Memory
- Language (speaking and understanding the spoken and written word)
- Perceptual–motor skills (organizing sequences of action correctly, such as in using eating utensils, putting on one's clothing, and identifying objects and people correctly by sight)
- Executive function (planning ahead, acting in socially appropriate ways, and thinking abstractly/hypothetically)
- Social cognition, which involves the processing of other people's faces and facial expressions, their voices, their posture, making judgments about others' personalities and motives, predicting their likely

behavior, and planning one's own interactions with others (Adolphs, 2005)

- Attention (maintaining sustained, focused attention over a period of time)

These abilities or skills are assessed in clinics via the use of standard neuropsychological tests. Although the tests are often used as outcome measures in clinical trials to determine the efficacy of a particular drug, what people are able to do in everyday life may be different from what they do on the tests. That is, deficits seen in certain areas of thinking on tests may not be mirrored in everyday life situations. At the same time, however, the tests may, in some cases, mirror quite well what people do in everyday life.

For example, a person may have memory problems revealed by the tests and also may, in everyday life, ask the same questions repeatedly even though the questions have been answered each time they were asked. The person may not recall having asked the question and may not recall the answer given. The same person may have trouble naming objects—may fail to recall the names of the objects and refer to this or that object instead as "that thing," for example. Conversely, a person may be unable to perform what is called a "three-stage command" (e.g., "Take this piece of paper, fold it in half, and put it on the floor") in the clinical testing situation but may be quite able to perform a three-stage command in an everyday life situation (e.g., "Please do me a favor and go over to Frank, pick up his lunch tray, and empty it in the trash can").

Executive function may also be affected depending on whether or not the frontal areas of the person's brain have suffered damage. This means that the person may not be able to plan ahead as he or she once did; may say things that are socially unacceptable (e.g., uttering profanities), whereas in earlier days this person would never do so publically; and may act inappropriately in other ways, such as walking about the house unclothed, whereas in earlier days the person would never do such a thing.

Why are there differences in performance on standard tests versus in everyday life?

There can be many reasons for these differences. One reason is that the standard neuropsychological tests administered in the clinic are "decontextualized." This means that people are asked questions or are asked to do certain things out of the blue, as it were, rather than in the typical social situations that we experience every day. For instance, on the Boston Naming Test, the person might be shown a drawing of a wristwatch and asked to name it. Now, there is nothing wrong with doing this, and most people can name this object easily. The person with dementia, however, may not be able to recall the word for that object when asked in that manner, when being put on the spot abruptly, as it were. The same person, however, in an everyday situation might see a friend's wristwatch and admire it by saying, "That's a lovely wristwatch you have on." In the natural social situation—in a typical dynamic social context— the person correctly names the object, but in the testing situation, which is not a typical everyday social context, he or she does not. At the same time, the person who cannot name the object may not be able to *recall* the word for the object but might know what the object is and can *recognize* the word if given a multiple-choice format. For example, I gave the Boston Naming Test to a woman diagnosed with a vascular dementia because she had incurred a number of small strokes. This test involves showing the person line drawings of different objects and the person has to name the objects. One of the black-and-white drawings I showed her was a stalk of asparagus. She looked at the drawing and said, "They're green, they're delicious, I love them, and they're too expensive." When I gave her some choices, she rejected the incorrect choices immediately and instantly chose "asparagus" when I said the word. Thus, the woman knew what she was looking at, could not recall the correct word, but could recognize it immediately upon hearing it spoken. So she did know what the name of this object was but could not recall it when asked on the test. If she truly did not know the name of the object, she would have been unable to choose the correct name upon hearing it, while rejecting the incorrect names quickly.

A second reason for the differences between what happens in the clinical testing situation and everyday life is that some people become extremely nervous when they go to a clinic. For example, many people, whether or not they have a diagnosis of dementia, have "white coat syndrome" such that when they visit the physician or dentist, they experience heightened anxiety and increases in blood pressure. Heightened anxiety can cause deficits in our ability to perform all sorts of tasks and can therefore interfere with our performance on standard tests. For example, 2 years before I met a woman diagnosed with AD, a neuropsychologist tested her in a hospital clinic. In his report, the neuropsychologist noted that she entered his office with an unsteady gait consistent with *apraxia* (an inability to perform skilled movements) and damage in the frontoparietal cortex of the brain. Alzheimer's disease is a degenerating illness and so in the very best of circumstances, it would have been just as bad when I met her as it was when the neuropsychologist tested her and reported her unsteady gait 2 years earlier. That is, people with AD do not get better with time. As it turned out, she and I took "power walks" together and she routinely left me almost exhausted. Indeed, her husband said, "She can walk me under the table." Her gait was anything but "unsteady." Therefore, the unsteadiness in her walking into the neuropsychologist's office was not due to AD and associated brain damage but, rather, due to her tremendous anxiety at the moment. The neuropsychologist's attribution of her unsteady gait to AD was an example of what social psychologists call the "fundamental attribution error" (Jones & Harris, 1967). This phenomenon refers to the tendency in Western culture to assume, for example, that people act as they do because of something about them—their disposition, their mentality—rather than because of the social situations in which they find themselves. So in this case, the neuropsychologist, looking for deficits due to AD, saw the woman's unsteady gait as she entered his office and attributed that to her illness rather than to the fact that she was extremely nervous in that situation.

A third reason for such discrepancies is that the attitude and demeanor of the person administering the tests can affect the person's ability to answer questions. Some examiners may be calm, warm, and encouraging, whereas others may be far less engaging and be distant from the person being tested. In both cases, people with dementia will react to the attitude of the examiner, and that will affect how well they respond to test questions. Usually, people respond better to examiners who are calm, warm, and encouraging than they do to examiners who are more distant and "objective."

For all these reasons, it is very important to recognize that standard tests may or may not (sometimes both) reveal what a person can and cannot do in terms of a number of cognitive abilities. Having said all this, it is still very important to note that decrements on clinical tests can reveal serious difficulties that must be acknowledged and accepted as being part of the diagnostic procedure. Whether or not all these difficulties or decrements are revealed in the same way in everyday life is a different question, and even though people may function more efficiently and effectively in everyday life than they do on the tests, they still ought to be able to answer most of the test questions without much difficulty. The main point here is that although the difficulties on the tests are real, the ability of people diagnosed with dementia to think clearly in everyday life situations should not be assumed to be an exact mirror of what they have done on the tests. In other words, we should not treat the person diagnosed *as if* his or her ability to think and understand is no greater than what the tests purport to demonstrate.

For example, the woman with the unsteady gait was said to have severe decrements in her ability to think conceptually given her performance on tests of "concept formation." In her association with me, she showed a very clear ability to conceive of and act upon the concept of fairness. She was honor bound not to do anything that she considered unfair to another person. This is a very important point to which I return later, because how we, who are deemed healthy, treat the person diagnosed can be extremely important: It can either help the person do things more easily or it can hinder what the person does and tries to do. As well, our expectations regarding the diagnosed person will affect what he or she actually does and how we interpret what the person does. This last point was exemplified clearly in the situation of the woman whose gait was "unsteady" and assumed to be so due to AD—the neuropsychologist interpreted what he saw based mainly on what he expected to see. It is unfortunate that all too often, the professionals who administer the tests and interview people in the clinics rarely, if ever, see the same people in natural social situations outside the clinic. This is especially true in the United States, where specialists such as geriatric psychiatrists rarely, if ever, go to their patients' homes. In the United Kingdom, however, this is not the case, for old-age psychiatrists frequently visit their patients at home.

Does the person diagnosed reveal deficits consistently?

Not necessarily. One of the hallmarks of brain damage is that there can be a great deal of variability in performance of this or that task or this or that skill—far more variability than was seen in the same person in healthier times. This variability can be from day to day, from hour to hour, and even moment to moment. Thus, in one moment, the person may be able to answer a question well, but in the next moment or next hour, the person may fail to do so.

What does this mean for care partners?

This kind of variability has to be understood as normal, meaning "usual," given the circumstances of brain injury. It can serve as something of an ally and can also be somewhat disturbing, depending on the point of view of the care partner. For example, knowing that there will be variability in a person's ability to find the correct word for an object or the name of a relationship (wife, husband, daughter, son, etc.) may be helpful to a care partner because it can lead him or her to encourage the person diagnosed by saying, "It'll come to you, so try to stay calm; pressuring yourself won't help." In this way, variability can be an ally because failure to do something correctly at one moment may not mean failure at all moments. When I say it may be disturbing to a care partner, I mean that when the person diagnosed does something correctly, it might lead the care partner to assume that things are getting better. When, in the next hour, the person diagnosed does the same thing incorrectly, it can lead the care partner to feel upset. So as long as it is clear that variability is the steady, or constant state, one need not misinterpret its meaning.

At times, spousal or adult-child care partners will question their spouse or parent about particular matters, such as the case of one man who, along with his wife who was diagnosed with AD, was being interviewed and filmed as part of a research project. The man asked his wife suddenly, "Who am I?" His wife could not say his name or "my husband" and laughed nervously while smiling warmly. The husband repeated the question a number of times, and his wife reacted in the same way, smiling all the while, until she finally said, "Oh, you're my best one" with great affection in her facial expression and her voice. It was clear that she simultaneously knew that he was a very special person to her and that she could not find the word "husband" or his name in that moment in that situation. Often, however, when not confronted that way, people with dementia may be able to recall the name or relationship noun. It is generally much more difficult for the person diagnosed (as well, oftentimes, for those not diagnosed) to recall information when "confronted," when put on the spot, than it is when the information in question is part of a natural conversation.

Why care partner and not caretaker?

If we return to the previous idea that what a person with dementia does in clinical testing situations can be affected by the attitude and demeanor of the examiner, we can begin understanding why it is crucial for us to be sensitive to the way we refer to the individuals who are trying to help the person with dementia and how they refer to themselves.

First, we must recognize that people with dementia are aware of how others treat them and can react appropriately in kind. We explore this idea more fully in a subsequent chapter. For now, though, if we think of ourselves as "caretakers," it is very easy to think of ourselves as doing things for the person diagnosed, and that can easily lead to wanting to do those things expeditiously. So, for example, in a very expensive nursing home in the mid-Atlantic area of the United States, a very well-meaning aide routinely fed an 85-year-old woman diagnosed with AD. The woman in question was fully capable of feeding herself, as she demonstrated consistently when encouraged by her granddaughter who was visiting her. Why did the aide feed the woman? It took less time than it would if the woman fed herself, mealtime was at a set hour, the aide had much to do, and time was of the essence because the aide's job performance depended on him or her doing everything on the list of things to do for residents in his or her charge. The aide was functioning as a caretaker, someone who is helping to "manage the AD patient." At the same time, the aide was creating a situation in which the woman with AD became increasingly less active in doing for herself what she always did and still could do for herself. That is, the aide was *disempowering* the woman and essentially treating her as if she were incapable or, perhaps, as if she were a child. The aide functioned as a caretaker, not helping the woman to help herself, not helping the woman to maximize her abilities, and, in the process, unwittingly increasing the woman's dependence further.

On the other hand, a care partner, caregiver, or carer (in the United Kingdom) is one half of an interactive relationship between two people wherein the aide, in this case, works to help the person with AD retain and use all of his or her abilities to the fullest degree. The two people work together with the goal being to engage the person with AD as a person rather than as a patient. If the person with AD eats slowly, perhaps that is the way it works best for him or her. No one should prevent a person from feeding him- or herself simply because it is not convenient for the person deemed healthy or the schedule of the nursing home. We spend decades of adult life choosing when to eat and how quickly to do so. Some people eat quickly, others eat slowly by comparison. Imagine how you would feel if someone said you must finish eating in a certain amount of time as if you were playing the old television program, "Beat the Clock." In another case, how would you would feel if, at 7:30 one morning, someone (an aide) told you it was time to take a shower and you really did not want to do so at that moment, being that you were still half asleep, but the aide insisted and began to pull you out of bed. This actually happened to someone I knew who was diagnosed with dementia and living in an expensive nursing home. The man in question, a retired Army general, at first said he did not want to take a shower at that time. The aide insisted and the retired general resisted. The aide tried to pull the retired general out of bed, and the general fought back and pushed the aide away. In doing so, the general became, in the words of the aide, "combative" and "uncooperative." The aide was not functioning as a care partner but, rather, as a caretaker whose job it was to make sure that the "dementia patient's" hygiene was taken care of at that time. To be fair, it is clear that the aide was simply trying to do his job even in a good-natured way at first. At the same time, the way the nursing home was set up required the aide to act as he did, so the aide is not alone in being at fault here. The problem was the philosophy of the nursing home administration that views caretaking as its responsibility and requires expeditious accomplishment of its goals. Must the care in a nursing home be provided in this way, or is there another way? I take up this question in a subsequent chapter.

Being a care partner is entirely different. It involves a vastly different system in a nursing home, and this entails an entirely different view of the person with dementia: The individual is a person first, who happens to have a diagnosis of dementia. As a result, the person may not be able to do things as quickly as in previous days. If one of the principal goals is to support the person's ability to act independently, then there needs to be an allowance for the increased time it takes for the person to feed him- or herself. The aide's role, the administration's role, the spousal care partner's role, and the adult-child care partner's role is to facilitate where facilitation is needed, to encourage independence whenever possible, and to respect the individual's needs to be independent and to retain self-respect. Care partners recognize that they are working *together*, whereas caretakers do what they need to do in whatever way is required. Care partners work *with* each other. Caretakers focus on accomplishing the task at hand. Care partners are people and relationship oriented. Caretakers are task oriented.

This distinction is illustrated beautifully in a study by Weaks et al. (2009) carried out in Scotland. Experienced Community Mental Health nurses were given person-centered, psychosocial counseling training. The nurses were unanimous in their praise for the program. They reported that as a result of the training, they shifted from "managing the patient" to "listening to and hearing their clients," from "working on their patients" to "working with their clients." They learned to listen to their clients, the people diagnosed with dementia, and to facilitate the expression of their clients' emotional needs and reactions. They went from being task-oriented to being person-oriented. In other words, they no longer viewed their job as telling their patients what to do, going through their checklists of tasks to perform with great efficiency, before moving on to the next "patient" they had to visit. Rather, they viewed their job as taking the time to listen to and understand the needs of their clients and those of family care partners, even if it meant that they did not check off every item on their list of things to do. They reported that they became more open and more vulnerable, that they listened more attentively to their clients, and that they became more personal than before the training. For example, one participant in the study said,

> I find that when I go out to see someone now I am not just looking at the form filling, the medicine. . . . I used to go in and think, "right—I have to get this form filled out and make sure I've got the right medication, you know, and out the door as quickly as possible to get to the next one." I am not doing that anymore. I am going in without any paper or pen or anything, you know, and I just sit and listen and it's amazing what you get from people just by not saying an awful lot, just nodding, just using counseling skills basically. (p. 14)

Another participant spoke of how this shift in approach affected her: "I find it difficult, very, very difficult and painful sometimes . . . but in terms of the relationship it takes that one step further" (p. 15).

This shift is reminiscent of the shift from Martin Buber's (1937) notion of "I–It" relationships to "I–Thou" relationships. The former type of relationship is detached, cool, abstract, keeping a safe distance emotionally, what often is incorrectly called "professional" these days, and what characterized the nurses' interactions with their "patients" before they received training. The latter relationships, on the other hand, involve moving toward the other person, being vulnerable and spontaneous, and this is precisely what the nurses reported experiencing with their clients after having gone through the program of training. They were more able to help their clients help themselves and find creative ways of maintaining certain important aspects of their lives. Interestingly, the nurses in the study by Weaks et al. (2009) reported that the skills they learned to use with people with dementia and their families were applicable to other situations in their lives and that they became more competent in their jobs and more confident in themselves as a result. So learning to be more attentive and more humane in their treatment of their clients and their clients' families allowed the nurses to become more humane in general.

This finding has been supported in a year-long study by Wendy Moyle and colleagues (2016), who compared the value of a capabilities model of dementia care with the usual and customary long-term care approach in four nursing homes in Australia. They examined the different models of care as they affected staff's experiences in their work and attitudes toward people diagnosed with dementia. As well, they studied the perceived quality of life of those diagnosed as reported by their family care partners. The capabilities model emphasizes 10 central human capabilities that include, but are not limited to,

1. feeling valued;
2. living independently with compassionate support from others;
3. experiencing and expressing emotion in ways true to oneself;
4. experiencing the best health possible;
5. planning for the future;
6. experiencing connection with others where one can contribute and be contributed to;
7. experiencing connection with others where there is self-respect and dignity and a shared humanity with others;
8. engaging nature as a natural part of living;
9. experiencing play that is personally meaningful and fun; and
10. experiencing control over one's life.

Staff members working with the capabilities model had improved attitudes toward working with people with dementia and reported better experiences in doing so. As well, working with this model rather than the usual long-term care model resulted in family members reporting that they perceived their loved ones to be enjoying a better quality of life. Thus, treating people with dementia in these very personalized ways led to greater job satisfaction for staff members and better living conditions for people diagnosed.

The clear implication of this admittedly small study is that a diagnosis of dementia does not prevent people from experiencing important aspects of life and responding positively to being treated in genuinely humane ways that they valued in their healthier days. In addition, staff people who engaged those important capabilities in people diagnosed were happier in their jobs as well. Thus, how we think about the person with dementia is very closely connected to the way we act toward him or her. If we believe that the person diagnosed is "an empty shell" or "demented," that will lead to what Buber (1937) called "I–It" relationships and "caretaker" approaches. If, however, we believe that the person diagnosed is a person first—albeit a person who has some significant losses in certain, but not all, mental and physical abilities—that will lead to what Buber called "I–Thou" relationships and "care partner" approaches that turn out to be far more satisfying and affirming for all concerned.

Does a diagnosis of dementia mean "the long goodbye"?

The answer is in two parts: (1) No, and (2) it can, but not necessarily. First, it is a fact that each of us is living with a death sentence from the moment we are born. We therefore hope that life itself from day one will entail a very long goodbye. So let us dispense with thinking about dementia as being the "long goodbye." To think of a diagnosis of dementia in these terms is to create a situation that is unhelpful to everyone concerned for reasons I discussed in the preceding section. Just the same, people often do what is unhelpful to them, so it is quite within the realm of possibility that people will view having a loved one diagnosed with dementia as "a long goodbye." Just the same, it does not have to be that way.

Instead, it could mean "The Long Hello," as author Cathie Borrie (2015) writes in her book by that name, describing her experience as a care partner to her mother, who was diagnosed with Parkinson's and Alzheimer's diseases. In this compelling book, Borrie comes to know her mother and reflect on their lives together in deeper, more compassionate, loving, helpful ways as a result of being her mother's care partner. The same was true for Elinor Fuchs (2005) as she discussed in her article in *The New York Times*. In the following excerpt, she recalls one particularly touching interaction with her mother:

> "Are you the one l-l-love?" she stammered on my last visit to her, her face lighting up with a little whoop of recognition. Of course, she could not summon the complex linkage among the woman before her, that woman's name, and the idea of "daughter." I didn't dwell on her failure to "know" me through names or roles. In the last act, we had found a new life together.

Clearly, these two women, Borrie and Fuchs, did not assimilate the rather drama-laden idea of dementia meaning "the long goodbye." Rather, they took it upon themselves to forge new relationships with their mothers—relationships that allowed for personal growth on everyone's part and for warm memories and loving hearts to develop right up to the end even though their mothers were diagnosed with dementia of the Alzheimer's type. It is one thing to note that it is possible to accomplish this, but it is another to learn exactly how they were able to do so. That is a subject I explore when I discuss the social aspects of AD.

Now that we have explored aspects of the syndrome called dementia, let us begin to explore the type of dementia that is caused by AD, for it causes the largest number of cases of dementia. Much of what we can learn about the Alzheimer's type of dementia can be applied to other types of dementia as well.

2

ALZHEIMER'S DISEASE

BIOLOGICAL ASPECTS

Alzheimer's disease (AD) was first identified by Alois Alzheimer in 1906 in his patient, Frau Auguste D. Dr. Alzheimer saw Frau D in 1901 and observed her rather striking symptoms that normally would have been described as "senile dementia." It would have been called this in her case as well, save for the fact that she was in her early 50s when Alzheimer saw her. She displayed severe memory dysfunction, problems speaking and understanding words (aphasia), an inability to perform skilled movements (apraxia), hallucinations (false perceptions), and delusions (false beliefs). Alzheimer performed a postmortem examination of her brain and found that it contained abnormal proteins (beta-amyloid plaques) and changes in neural structures (neurofilbrillary tangles inside neurons, or nerve cells). Although this was discovered in 1906 and named by Emil Kraepelin in 1910, AD was not given a great deal of attention for decades. Even as late as 1970, noted psychologist Brendan Maher commented in his book, *Principles of Psychopathology*, that AD was not found with any significant frequency in the population and was thus of little interest to psychopathology students. As a result of the significant increase in the life span of adults in the developed world, however, the incidence of AD has grown significantly, and AD has become of tremendous interest to health care professionals and nonprofessionals alike. Currently, AD affects 5.4 million people in the United

States, and 44 million worldwide have been diagnosed with AD or another dementia, with the vast majority of the cost of AD going to nursing home care and care at home (Hurd et al., 2013).

What does Alzheimer's disease do to the brain?

The plaques and tangles occur in the cortex, the outer layer of cells of the brain, and in a structure called the hippocampus, which is shaped like a seahorse, hence its name (from Greek). Plaques and tangles contribute to the death of the brain's nerve cells, called neurons, which transmit messages from place to place in the brain and throughout the body. These plaques and tangles are said to distinguish AD from other types of dementia, such as vascular dementia and Lewy body dementia. Vascular dementia is the result of blockages in blood vessels or bleeding in the brain (small strokes), both of which cause the death of neurons. Vascular dementia has a more sudden onset than does AD unless the strokes are very small and their effects accumulate, and it is not, by its nature, degenerative unless the person has additional strokes. Lewy body dementia and Parkinson's dementia are related as both have Lewy bodies, which are clumps of alpha synuclein proteins in neurons. In addition to problems with memory and executive functions, among the most common symptoms with Parkinson's disease dementia are problems such as tremor, stiffness, and difficulty walking. With Lewy body dementia, visual hallucinations occur. There are only two ways to determine if there are plaques of different sizes and shapes and tangles in the brain: biopsy and autopsy. Clearly, for reasons of safety, biopsies are rarely performed. There has been some controversy as to which protein is critical to AD. Some scientists believe that one type, the beta type outside of neurons, is critical, but others believe that the tau protein tangles inside neurons are critical (Whitehouse, 2008). Whatever the critical cause may be, and both may be critical, the result is the death of neurons, which thus results in the shrinkage of the brain and loss of various abilities that were mediated by those areas of the brain before they were damaged.

Is there a genetic component?

Important studies carried out in the 1990s and published by the National Institute on Aging (2003) investigated families who were thought to be at very high risk of developing AD. These studies revealed that there are rare genetic mutations on chromosome 21 that increase the formation of beta-amyloid proteins that ultimately destroy neurons. Other mutations have been found on chromosomes 1 and 14 and, like that on chromosome 21, cause a powerful genetic form of AD that has a 50 percent probability of being inherited from a parent. These mutations are extremely rare, with only a few thousand families affected, and those affected will develop young-onset symptoms. That these mutations are very rare does not, however, mean that their effects are not serious and tremendously challenging to the people affected and their families for many reasons, some unique to people with young-onset symptoms. These families can have blood tests that show whether they are carrying the gene that can result in the *familial* type of the disease.

There is another category of genetic risk that involves late-onset, so-called *sporadic* type of AD that is found in people aged 60 years or older. In these people, there is a variant of a gene on chromosome 19 that affects the production of *apolipoprotein E* (ApoE), of which there are three types (or alleles): E2, E3, and E4. If one inherits E4 from each parent, one will have the highest risk of developing late-onset AD. If one inherits E4 from only one parent, the risk is diminished. ApoE is a protein that normally helps transportation of cholesterol.

It is extremely important to note that even though the presence of ApoE-4 can increase one's susceptibility to AD, it *does not, by itself,* cause the disease. So if you have genetic testing done and find out that you have ApoE-4, it does not mean that you will inevitably develop AD. It means that the risk is greater than it would be otherwise. One of the problems that can occur after genetic testing indicates the presence of ApoE-4 was revealed by a student of mine who discussed her father's genetic test results and his reaction to them. The man was middle-aged and was told that his testing showed he had a 17 percent chance of developing AD in later life. His daughter noted that having heard this information, whenever her father could not immediately recall something, he began to wonder aloud, "Uh-oh, is this the beginning of AD?" Now, most of us as we grow older develop problems recalling immediately that which we could easily recall when we were in our twenties and thirties and forties, and this is not necessarily the harbinger of AD. It remains to be seen whether or not worry and other psychological states such as depression and feelings of stress have any effect on the development of AD in some people. In any case, that my student's father was so deeply concerned was not necessarily a good thing for him or for his family.

Does the existence of plaques and tangles in the brain mean that one has Alzheimer's disease?

Not necessarily. Blessed and colleagues (1968) and Tomlinson and colleagues (1968, 1970) conducted postmortem examinations of the brains of elderly people diagnosed with dementia and those who were not diagnosed. They found that 40 percent of the people diagnosed had no brain atrophy, and 46 percent of the nondiagnosed group had no cerebral atrophy (shrinkage due to the death of brain cells). With regard to senile plaques, 16 percent of those diagnosed did not have any, whereas 21 percent of those not diagnosed did not have any. In the case of neurofibrillary tangles, 28 percent of those diagnosed and 39 percent of those not diagnosed showed none. Other researchers, such as Albert and colleagues (1984), showed that cerebral atrophy is present in many, but not all, people diagnosed with dementia. So the presence of plaques and tangles does not necessarily mean that one has AD, and one can have these and still be asymptomatic.

Furthermore, no connection has been found between the numbers of plaques and tangles found and the degree of cognitive impairment demonstrated in people with AD. Often, people with levels of plaques that are above and beyond what is considered defining of AD do as well on cognitive tests as do people with low levels of plaques. All in all, the presence of beta-amyloid plaques in the brain does not mean that the person has or will have AD at some point later in life (Whitehouse, 2008). Plaques may begin forming in our brains even in our twenties, so it is quite common for older people to have them in their brains. Knopman and colleagues (2003) found that almost 33 percent of people who are asymptomatic have enough amyloid plaques in their brains that they would have been diagnosed with AD if they had demonstrable symptoms. So it is very difficult, if not impossible, to assume that the presence of many beta-amyloid plaques means that a person has AD.

Indeed, a now famous study called the Nun Study, conducted by Snowden and discussed further in his 1997 article, showed just how little we really know about the relationship between plaques and tangles and AD. A group of 678 American members of the School of Sisters of Notre Dame religious order was studied for decades. Their writing from when they were in their twenties was examined and compared with their memory abilities as they grew older, and when they died, their brains were examined carefully. Sister Mary, one of the nuns in the study, taught full-time until she was 77 years old and part-time until she retired at age 84 years. Even after that, she continued to live in the convent and gave important lessons on the subject of aging with grace, remained a student of current events in the world, and was an avid reader. She signed up to donate her brain to research, and after she died, her brain was examined and was found to contain a large number of plaques and tangles consistent with AD. Yet, when she was 101 years old, her score on the Mini-Mental State Exam, which is frequently used to assess thinking ability, was 27 out of a possible 30, putting her in the normal range. Interestingly, given her age and rather poor formal education, her score was predicted by the researchers to be 11 based on her education and 8 based on her age. According to Snowden, it may have been the case that Sister Mary's significant abilities were due to the location of the plaques and tangles in her brain. There are many unknowns yet to be solved in terms of understanding what factors may accompany the presence of plaques and tangles in the brain so as to yield the outward symptoms of AD.

What causes plaques to develop at all?

It is unclear what causes the development of beta-amyloid, and its significance for the symptoms of AD is not well understood. The development of plaques and tangles may be a consequence of aging (Giannakopoulos et al., 1995; Stam, Wigboldus, & Smeulders, 1986). So again, if normal (meaning "usual") aging involves the development of these changes in the brain and people can live with these without showing symptoms of decline as in AD, what is it that makes AD happen? It is not clear to this day exactly what makes AD happen, and this is one of the important puzzles that researchers seek to solve.

How is Alzheimer's disease diagnosed?

There is no test that can reveal with certainty that a person has AD. The most that physicians can say is that someone has "probable AD." This is true for a number of reasons:

1. As mentioned previously, plaques and tangles may be numerous in the brain, but the person may not show symptoms of dementia.
2. Some people may have fewer plaques and tangles and yet have stronger symptoms of dementia.

3. As people grow older, they may have had or have vascular problems or other abnormalities in the brain in addition to plaques and tangles. As a result, there are many so-called mixed dementias because some people have a number of different abnormalities in their brains.
4. There is no one single biological identifier that is consistent in every person diagnosed with AD.

In general, the diagnosis of probable AD is made by "exclusion." That is, other possible causes of dementia must be ruled out first. Among these are vascular problems such as strokes, vitamin deficiencies (including B vitamins), normal pressure hydrocephalus, depression, brain tumors, head trauma such as concussions, Parkinson's disease, delirium, HIV, meningitis, syphilis, chronic alcoholism, and others. This means that you cannot be diagnosed with probable AD after a visit to your internist or general practitioner who notes that you have memory problems. Extensive testing and examinations must be done first, and these are often best done in a reputable hospital (often a university hospital) by a team of health professionals. Also, as noted previously, even then the best that the professionals can provide is a diagnosis of "probable AD." For convenience, I do not use "probable" in the balance of this book, but you should understand that "probable" is implied throughout.

When a person has AD, he or she shows signs of losses and/or changes in certain abilities compared to those same abilities in healthier days. The losses are gradual, not sudden. Some losses and/or changes occur due to damage in the brain. Other changes and/or losses can occur for psychological and social reasons.

Are there some other biomarkers that can be used for diagnosing probable Alzheimer's disease?

Yes. They include the following: elevated tau and phosphor tau protein and decreased levels of beta-amyoid 42 in the person's cerebrospinal fluid, positive positron emission tomography

(PET) scan of the brain showing amyloid, and "disproportionate" brain atrophy in the temporal lobes of the brain, as well as in the medial areas of the parietal lobe cortex as seen on magnetic resonance imaging (MRI) scans. But these biomarkers are not suggested for routine diagnostic purposes as yet (McKhann et al., 2011). McKhann and co-authors present the most updated account of the diagnostic approaches to "probable AD" as well as "possible AD."

In the following sections, I discuss those changes that occur due to brain damage alone. In subsequent chapters, I discuss alterations that can occur due to psychological and social reasons. This is why I have taken a "biopsychosocial" approach to what everyone needs to know about AD.

What sorts of memory problems are caused by Alzheimer's disease?

I phrase the question this way because AD does not cause problems with all types of memory functions. There are different types of memory and different ways to retrieve information from memory. AD causes problems with some but not all, so we have to be specific in answering this question so that care partners are able to recognize their loved one's strengths as well as weaknesses in this important area.

Care partners often note that their loved one who has been diagnosed with AD repeatedly asks the same questions even though the questions have been answered each time. The person with probable AD seems not to recall (1) the answer that has been given and (2) that he or she asked that same question before. This person is having trouble retrieving information from memory via the process of *recall*. You can distinguish between recall and *recognition*, another way to retrieve information from memory, through the following examples: We use recall when we are asked questions such as What day of the week is this? What city are we in? When is your birthday? What are the names of your children? and What were your parents' first names? If you were taking an exam and objective questions required you to fill in the blank space, you would be using recall to find the word or words that go in the blank. Recall is the most difficult of the various methods of retrieval from memory, and it becomes more difficult as we age, even if we do not have a diagnosis of AD or another type of dementia. So just because you experience more difficulty in using recall at the age of 60 years than you did at age 40 years, it does not mean that you are experiencing the onset of AD.

Recognition is another method of retrieving information from memory. A common situation in which we, as students, use recognition is taking a multiple-choice examination. Here, the correct answer is given to us among other possibilities, and we have to pick it out correctly—so we are recognizing the correct answer when we see or hear it presented. This method of retrieval is easier than recall, and it can function well even if recall is problematic. So if you have a loved one diagnosed with probable AD who has problems recalling information, you might help him or her by using the multiple-choice format. Instead of asking, "What did you have for lunch?" ask, "Did you have fish for lunch?" and provide other possibilities as well if the answer to this question is "no."

One of the structures in the brain that is affected by AD rather early in the progress of the disease is the *hippocampus*. As with most other brain structures, we have two of them, one in each hemisphere. The hippocampus is especially involved in a type of memory called *explicit memory*, of which recall and recognition are the methods of retrieval that are used. When the hippocampus is damaged, we have difficulty retrieving information about recent events via recall especially. That is why the person with AD asks the same question repeatedly even though it has been answered previously each time the question was posed. The person is not trying to be difficult or annoy his or her interlocutor but, rather, truly cannot recall that he or she already asked the question and that the question was answered. This problem is a direct result of brain injury especially in the hippocampus.

Sometimes, the problem with recall reveals itself when the person with AD cannot find the correct words he or she wants to use. That is, the person cannot *recall* the word or words in question. Professionals often refer to this phenomenon as "word-finding problems." Often, the person will refer to this or that object as "that thing" rather than using the correct noun because recall of the particular noun is compromised. This kind of problem can be exacerbated if we "confront" the person with AD by asking him or her directly, sometimes out of the blue, "What do you call this object?" while pointing to the object or to a drawing or photo of the object. Thus, the person with AD might not be able to recall the word "spoon" when shown a drawing of a spoon on a test (e.g., the Boston Naming Test) and asked to name the object. That same person might, while sitting at the dinner table, having been served soup, point to a spoon on the table and ask someone, "Can you please pass me that spoon?" What this shows is that there can be, and often is, a major difference between what people with AD or another dementia do on clinical tests and what they do in everyday life situations. As noted in Chapter 1, however, there can be great variability in that same person's ability to name the object called a spoon both in everyday life and in clinical testing situations, so the person might ask for the spoon clearly at one moment and then 10 minutes later, having dropped the spoon, might say, "Oh, I just dropped the, the, uh, the thing. May I have another, please?"

Taking this issue of finding words a bit further, it is important to understand that even though a person with AD or another dementia may not be able to recall a particular word, that does not mean that he or she has forgotten the word or that the word has been somehow erased from the person's mental lexicon. An example of this phenomenon can demonstrate as well the difference between recall and recognition and how the former might be compromised when the latter is still working. I was having a conversation with a woman diagnosed with probable AD, Dr. M (Sabat, 2001, p. 77) and she said,

"I happened to have a visit to my, uh ... uh ... (12 seconds elapse) ... the person who takes care of me when I have any problem physically."

I asked, "A dentist?" "No, not in this case," she replied.

I asked, "A physician?" She replied, "Yes."

Here, she could not recall the word she sought but instead used a different way to indicate what she was trying to communicate. Professionals call this "circumlocution" because the person is essentially talking "around" the word. I thought I knew the word she was failing to recall at the moment, and so I asked her questions in a multiple-choice way and she *recognized* the word she sought when she heard it, after already having rejected another possibility that I presented to her. So here we see that she still had the word in her mental lexicon, as it were, and even though she could not recall it, she could recognize it when she heard it spoken. So the brain damage that prevented her from recalling the word she sought did not deprive her of the ability to recognize it when it was presented to her. It is of great importance that care partners realize that not being able to recall something in this case, and in many others, does not mean that it is forgotten. In other words, (1) remembering is more than just recalling, and (2) not being able to recall something does not mean that that something has been forgotten. One cannot recognize the correct word or words if one has truly forgotten them.

Can we mistake word-finding problems for more serious pathology in a person with Alzheimer's disease?

Often, family care partners experience troubling moments such as the following: The person with AD refers to her daughter as her mother. Does the person with AD really believe that the young woman standing before her is her mother, who has been deceased for decades? I have heard people in this situation say that their mother is having hallucinations, does not know the difference between her mother and her daughter, or "does not know who I am anymore" or some other variant of this troubling state of affairs.

A different, perhaps more parsimonious, way to analyze this situation is to consider other possibilities:

1. The mother is calling the woman who is her daughter her mother because her daughter is taking care of so many things for her that it feels as though her daughter has become a person who is acting like her mother—who is "mothering" her, so to speak.
2. The mother is having word-finding problems and cannot recall the word "daughter" and so she is using another noun that denotes a female member of the immediate family.
3. Not using the correct noun in this case does not mean that the mother does not know who her daughter is anymore.

It may be helpful to care partners to keep these possibilities in mind so as to avoid assuming that a psychiatric problem exists when a far less troubling situation may be occurring.

Frankly, at some point, does it really matter which noun the elder person uses if there is a loving relationship being experienced? One possibly helpful example that I mentioned previously is that of the husband asking his wife, who has been diagnosed with probable AD, "Who am I?" At first, she laughs, and he asks again. She laughs again, a bit more nervously, but still does not answer. He persists further and repeats the question again, and she finally laughs and says with great warmth in her voice, "Oh, you're my best one." Clearly, she knows who he is, that he is a very special person to her, even though she cannot recall his name or the noun "husband" in that moment.

There may come a point in the progress of the disease that a person with AD not only cannot recall a loved one's name or relationship but also may show no outward signs whatsoever of recognizing the loved one, and this would be deeply distressing for most of us. Just the same, that does not mean that we cannot continue to do our best to love and honor the relationship that we know we recognize. An apocryphal story illustrates this point. A man visited his wife, who had been diagnosed with probable AD, every day in the nursing home where she resided. He told friends and acquaintances that she no longer seemed to know who he was. One day, he was late in going to visit her and was hurrying along when a friend asked him why he was rushing so much, given that she did not know who he is. He replied, "But I know who *she* is."

Does the person with Alzheimer's disease have "memory loss" or is it "memory dysfunction"?

The mass media as well as staff members in nursing homes and day centers and even the website of the Alzheimer's Disease Association frequently refer to one of the symptoms of AD as "memory loss." Indeed, all seem to equate a failure to *recall* with forgetting. But what does "memory loss" actually mean? It could mean a number of things, including the following:

1. The erasure of memories of past and recent events
2. The erasure of memories of recent events primarily
3. The inability to make new memories so that recent events never become encoded by the brain and thus are not there to retrieve

In order to analyze these possibilities, it is important that we distinguish between two types of memory/two types of retrieval from memory:

1. Explicit memory
2. Implicit memory

Explicit memory involves the conscious retrieval of specific information such as recent events via either of the two methods discussed previously: recall and recognition. In each of these cases, the questioner is asking directly for a particular piece of information, and there is generally only one correct answer. So if the question is "What did you have for lunch today?" there is only one correct answer and a tremendous number of possible incorrect answers. The same holds true for a question such as "What's my name?" or "Who am I?" As we have seen, it is possible for a person with probable AD to fail to recall the answers to such questions while simultaneously recognizing the correct answer when it is presented among a series of incorrect choices. Both ways of asking the questions are quite direct. There is another kind of memory called implicit memory, and knowing about it is extremely important to everyone concerned—those diagnosed and their care partners as well.

What is implicit memory?

Implicit memory is inferred (the existence of a memory is implied) from a change in a person's performance or behavior as a result of previous experience that the person may deny, or not recall, having had. Thus, the person may not be able to recollect consciously some previous experience, but his or her actions will reflect a memory of that previous experience nonetheless because different brain systems are involved in implicit and explicit memory (Howard, 1991; Schacter, 1987; Squire, 1994). One experimental, laboratory illustrated, example of this phenomenon is a word-stem completion task. A person with a memory dysfunction, such as Korsakoff's syndrome or AD, is presented with a list of words to study including the word DEFEND. The person's memory of the words on the list can be tested in different ways. In one format, testing explicit memory, the person can be given the word stem DEF and then asked to fill in the blank so as to make a word that he or she studied on the list presented previously. In another format, testing implicit memory, the person would be asked to complete the blank so as to form the first word that comes to mind. Note that in this latter format, there is no mention of the list of words presented previously. When employing the first format, using explicit memory, it is not uncommon for the person with AD or Korsakoff's syndrome to respond by saying, "What list?" By asking this question, the person diagnosed with AD or Korsakoff's syndrome exhibits a dysfunction in explicit memory, specifically recall. The same person who appears to have no memory of having studied the list of words will then complete the word stem correctly if asked to fill in the blank so as to make the first word that comes to mind. When one realizes that there are many words that begin with DEF, it becomes apparent that a person could not simply be "lucky" in guessing correctly.

Such findings were noted in people with AD in the early stages three decades ago (Morris & Kopelman, 1986) and in the mild to moderate stages as well (Dick, Kean, & Sands, 1989; Grosse, Wilson, & Fox, 1990; Partridge, Knight, & Feehan, 1990; Perani et al., 1993; Randolph, Tierney, & Chase, 1995; Russo & Spinnler, 1994). In the late 1990s, Fleischman et al. (1997) showed intact word-stem completion priming in people with AD, even though the subjects had poor recognition (explicit memory) of the material presented previously. To be fair, there is some inconsistency in the literature about this type of learning in people with AD (Spaan, Raaijmakers, & Jonker, 2003), and further research is required to explore fully the reasons for the inconsistencies. Often, however, people with AD have been able to learn and retrieve information correctly in an implicit memory task even though they were unable to do so when tested via an explicit memory task.

Do people diagnosed with probable Alzheimer's disease show intact implicit memory in everyday life?

Yes. A few case examples are illustrative. Mr. C (Sabat, 2006) always mowed the lawn and trimmed the shrubs around the family home. He continued doing so after having been diagnosed with probable AD in the mild to moderate stages. Even though he never had any mishaps, Mrs. C thought it might be dangerous for her husband to continue to mow the lawn. She put a padlock on the shed in which the lawnmower and other tools were kept. Mr. C, finding the shed locked, broke the padlock, retrieved the lawnmower, and mowed the lawn. Feeling even more anxious and without discussing this course of action with her husband, Mrs. C arranged with John, the oldest of their three adult children, to take the lawnmower. When the grass needed cutting again, Mr. C went to the shed and found the lawnmower missing and reported to his wife that it had been stolen. At this point, she finally explained that she and John agreed that it might be dangerous for Mr. C to use the lawnmower and that John agreed to take it to his house.

Five days later, the adult children came home for Sunday dinner and Mr. C greeted the two younger children warmly with hugs and kisses. When John arrived, however, Mr. C uncharacteristically ignored him completely. When Mrs. C asked if he was angry with John, Mr. C replied, "Yeah." When asked why, he replied, "I don't know." Mr. C had not, previous to this occasion, behaved in such a way toward John. Thus, Mr. C made a memory of his wife and son "conspiring" to prevent him from using the lawnmower to perform a job that he enjoyed and gave him a sense of purpose. He was very upset by this, feeling that he was ignored in the process and not even given the opportunity to discuss this situation with the rest of the family. Thus, he felt disrespected, hurt, and angry. That he made a memory of his feeling and its relationship to John is implied (hence implicit memory) by his uncharacteristic angry reaction to John 5 days after having learned about what became of the lawnmower. Because his explicit memory system involving the hippocampus was damaged due to AD, he could not recall the details of why he was angry with John, but he did have an intact memory *that* he was angry with John. So what is "lost" is the memory of the exact details, but there is still a memory of the feeling and its connection to John.

Therefore, Mr. C's experience was not erased entirely. He was righteously indignant about how he was treated. Thus, we see that Mr. C did not have "memory loss" but, rather, "memory dysfunction" because he made a new memory of how he felt in connection with John but was unable to recall the details of the experience that inspired his feelings.

Another example is that of Mrs. L, who was diagnosed with probable AD and who was a participant at an adult day center. She had always been gregarious, kind, and service-oriented. When she was tested formally with a battery of clinical tests, among the tasks she could not complete was a three-stage (or three-step) command: "Take this piece of paper, fold it in half, and put it on the floor." At the day center, it was a different story, however. One day, as people were finishing their lunch, I said to Mrs. L, "Would you do me a favor please?" She smiled immediately and nodded. I then said, "Would you go over to Frank (another participant seated at the lunch table), pick up his tray, and empty it into the trash can, please?" Note that this is a three-stage command. She immediately did exactly that, thereby showing that the context in which one asks someone to do something is very important. What is more important for our present purpose, however, is what happened 2 days later when I returned to the day center. Lunch was coming to an end and Mrs. L, with no prompting at all, approached me and asked, "Do you have something for me to do?" I said, "Like what?" She replied, "I don't know." Mrs. L made a memory of me having asked her to do something that she seemed to have found pleasurable because she was being of service. Her explicit memory system, being damaged, did not allow her to recall the exact details of what it was that I asked her to do. Just the same, her implicit memory system was still intact and so she made a memory of something connected to me, as was shown by her asking me if I had something for her to do. Prior to this occasion, she had never asked me anything resembling the question, "Do you have something for me to do?"

One final example involves Mrs. G, who was a member of a support group for people with AD for which I was co-leader for a number of years. I wanted to meet with her to interview her, and so we agreed that I would phone her to set up a time to meet. Speaking with her by phone, I suggested that we meet at the church where the support group met and that we should meet the next day at 10 a.m. She agreed.

We continued to converse for a few minutes when she interrupted and said, "So where and when are we going to meet?" Instead of saying, "What did I just tell you?" or "What did we just agree on about that?" I simply answered her question as if we had not yet agreed on a time and place. We continued to converse and after another few minutes, she asked again about when and where we would meet. Again, I treated her question as if it were the first time she asked. It would have done no good to tell her that we already spoke about that and had agreed on the time and place because clearly she did not recall that. This sequence of events repeated itself three or four more times. Finally, she said, "So what time are we going to meet?" I said, "Take a guess." She said, "Ten o'clock." I replied, "Exactly right."

Although she repeatedly asked about our meeting time and place, seemingly indicating that she had forgotten what I had told her five or six times, she still made a memory of the correct time. If I had said, "What time did we agree on?" it would have caused her great anxiety because she clearly did not recall that we had agreed on a time and place and that she had asked about it a number of times. The key in all this is *how you ask for the information*. That is, by asking, "What did I tell you?" you are engaging the person's explicit memory system. This means that the person has to recall a specific piece of information, and that is precisely what she could not do. If, however, I say, "Take a guess" instead, there are three advantages: (1) There is no pressure at all because one can always guess incorrectly without embarrassment, (2) there is no reference to my having already told her that information, and (3) I am tapping her implicit memory system. That Mrs. G guessed the time correctly is evidence of her intact implicit memory: She made a memory of the time at which we agreed to meet, but she could not *recall* that information when asked directly. When asked indirectly ("Take a guess"), she retrieved the information accurately. This was not at all a "lucky guess," as we can appreciate from the following logic:

1. If there were 12 daylight hours and we agreed to meet during the day, and we agreed further to meet on the hour, she would have had a 1 in 12 chance of guessing correctly.
2. But we could have agreed to meet on the half hour or the quarter hour as well.
3. Therefore, the odds against her guessing correctly were tremendous.
4. That she did so on the first attempt shows that she knew the time at which we agreed to meet, but she could not consciously recall that information or the fact that we had spoken about it previously.

Is treating each repetition of the same question as if it were the first time easy to do?

For me, it was rather easy, given what I knew and my relationship with Mrs. G, but it might not be nearly as easy for an adult child or spouse to respond this way for a number of reasons. First, such close relatives have strong, decades-old, emotional ties to the person with AD. To see a loved one "weakened" in this way, showing hallmark symptoms of AD, with all that they think it means, can be tremendously saddening, threatening, and can create in the care partner a deep sense of loss, of grief. Perhaps the care partner feels also that it is just not fair that this should happen to a loved one and no one wants to see this happen. As a result, a well-meaning care partner might lose control of his or her emotions and say, in a raised voice, something like, "What did I just tell you?" or "How many times do I have to repeat this information?"—neither of which does any good. So it can be a challenge to respond as I did, and it might take some concerted practice, but it is likely to be the best way for everyone concerned.

How can knowing about implicit memory be helpful to everyone?

If you do not understand that people with probable AD have intact implicit memory systems even though their explicit memory systems are damaged, you can make very unfortunate errors. For example, without an understanding of implicit memory, Mr. C's behavior toward his son was interpreted as being "irrational hostility," often mentioned as a sign of AD. The family assumed that Mr. C had no memory of his having been told that John had taken the lawnmower away because Mr. C could not state why he was angry with John. In other words, because he could not state why he was angry with his son, and because he had a diagnosis of AD, Mrs. C assumed that there was no reason for Mr. C's anger; hence, she viewed it as being "irrational." The existence of intact implicit memory systems allows us to understand Mr. C's reaction as "righteous indignation" and not "irrational hostility." Righteous indignation is not pathological. It is a healthy reaction to a perceived insult. Irrational hostility, however, is most certainly pathological. Therefore, dysfunctional explicit memory (faulty conscious recall or recognition) *does not mean* that people with AD cannot (1) learn new information, (2) retain what they learn for long periods of time, and (3) act on the basis of that new information or new experience. This knowledge can spell the difference between viewing the behavior of people with AD as pathological and viewing it as being rationally connected to their previous experiences, even if they cannot recall those experiences.

In addition, this knowledge allows care partners to understand that they should not do or say anything that could be hurtful to the person diagnosed because they think that the person with AD "won't remember it anyway." On the contrary, the person diagnosed *can make new memories*; therefore, it is even more important to treat him or her with common courtesy, respect, and sensitivity, given that the person diagnosed has already been negatively affected by brain damage resulting in memory dysfunction, language difficulties, organizing complex movements, and the like. Care partners must assume that their loved one who is diagnosed will be affected long term, having made implicit memories, by what they say and do. To do otherwise would be adding insult to injury, essentially pouring salt on an open wound.

Are there other dysfunctions that are caused by Alzheimer's disease-related brain damage?

Yes, there are quite a few, all of which are included in the syndrome called dementia. One dysfunction is called *visual agnosia*. Agnosia means "not to know," as is denoted by the term *agnostic*. In the case of visual agnosia, the person diagnosed can see clearly but has trouble naming what he or she is seeing—but this is not because the person cannot recall or recognize the word for the object. The person might be able to describe the object's various features but not be able to say what it is or even use it properly without naming it. Oliver Sacks's patient, Dr. P, who was diagnosed with AD, demonstrated an especially vivid example of visual agnosia (Sacks, 1985). On one occasion when he visited Dr. P, Sacks wore a red rose in the lapel buttonhole on his jacket. Sacks had already asked Dr. P to name some objects, including a sphere, a cube, and other so-called Platonic solids that are part of the neurological kit Sacks carried. Dr. P named all the solids correctly, including the dodecahedron, a 12-sided solid. Sacks then removed the rose from his lapel and handed it to Dr. P, who said, "About six inches in length, a convoluted red form with a linear green attachment." Sacks responded, "Yes, ... and what do you think it is, Dr. P?" Dr. P answered, "Not easy to say . . . it lacks the simple symmetry of the Platonic solids, although it may have a higher symmetry of its own. I think this could be an inflorescence or flower." Sacks then asked Dr. P to smell it and Dr. P said, "Beautiful! An early rose. What a heavenly smell" (pp. 12–13). Here, Dr. P did not have a word-finding problem because he identified the object correctly when he smelled it. When he looked at the rose, Dr. P saw and described only its various features, but he could not organize all those separate features into a unified whole object. Thus, a person with visual agnosia would not be able to use eating utensils properly because he or she would not appreciate by looking at these objects what they actually are. Likewise, a person with a visual agnosia would have difficulty getting dressed for the same reason. This condition arises because part of the person's brain, in what is sometimes referred to as the *association area* of the *occipital lobe* that is toward the rear of the brain, is damaged by the effects of AD. People with AD can also exhibit a very specific type of agnosia called *prosopagnosia*, wherein they have difficulties in recognizing familiar faces and learning to recognize new faces. Some people with this disorder cannot recognize their own faces, such as when looking in a mirror. Usually, the term prosopagnosia is used for those who have this condition but do not have other neurodegenerative disorders such as AD (Davies-Thompson, Pancaroglu, & Barton, 2014).

Another result of brain damage due to AD is a condition called *apraxia*. This is a disorder in which the person has difficulty organizing a sequence of movements in the correct order. The person has no paralysis, so movement per se is not a problem, but putting the sequence of movements together to achieve a goal is the problem. Thus, the person has difficulty tying shoelaces because that requires movements organized in a particular order to accomplish. The same holds true for putting on one's clothes, making a phone call, engaging in cursive writing, or imitating what others do. Apraxia is common in people with AD and can be seen to occur often after memory and language problems have existed for some time (Green et al., 1995). So the person in this case can name an object by sight, such as a shoe, can state what a shoe's purpose is and on which part of the body one would wear it, but cannot put the shoe on and tie the laces.

Still another condition that AD can cause is *aphasia*, a disorder of language. The expressive type involves dysfunctions in speaking or writing, whereas the receptive type involves dysfunctions in reading or understanding the spoken word. Specifically, there can be problems in the way the person with AD constructs sentences because they may not be syntactically correct, thereby making it more difficult for listeners to understand. Usually, people with AD do much worse on standardized tests of language function such as the Boston Diagnostic Aphasia Examination than they do in natural conversation in their familiar social world. Still, people can experience very troubling losses in the ability to read fluently and speak fluently in social situations. Speaking fluently can become even more problematic because people with AD experience difficulties in finding (recalling) the words they want to use. At times, they may also use the first few letters of a word correctly but then follow up with something other than the word they want to use. For example, Mr. K was a participant at an adult day center and was participating in a small group discussion about the merits of teaching young people in public schools about different religious traditions. Mr. K, a highly educated man, began by saying, "I think it would be adventurous for the children . . . it would be adventurous, I think that it would be adventurous . . . uh . . . uh . . . it would be *advantageous* for the children to learn about different religions." At first, he seemed to be stuck on the word "adventurous." As I listened to him, I thought, yes, it could be adventurous depending on the way the teacher went about organizing the lessons, but this word was not sitting well with me and apparently it was not sitting well with Mr. K either because he kept coming back to it. When he finally said "advantageous," he continued speaking the entire sentence he had begun and then went on to say more. So in this case, he spoke the correct first three letters, "adv," but could not at first find the word "advantageous" and said "adventurous" instead. He heard himself say "adventurous" and knew that that was not the word he wanted to use, and he kept repeating it, not wanting to continue the thought with a word other than the one that would convey his thought accurately. Either word would have conveyed his affirmative answer to the question, but "advantageous" was the word that was most accurate for him.

The same sort of phenomenon occurred in one of my conversations with Dr. M (Sabat, 2001) when she was discussing how her parents reacted when she left home at the tender age of 16 years, quite uncommon for women of her age at that time (the 1930s). Talking about her parents, she said, "And I got a place for my own . . . and then I said that I wanted to be with them sometime, but I didn't want to be with them all the time." I asked, "How did they take it?" She replied, "Well, my mother tried to get two kids, uh, who, who had, that she would take into the house in view, view of, of me. Not, not, in *view*—that's not the WORD!" (Her voice grew louder and louder.) I responded by saying, "I know . . . and I know what the word is. It sounds like view and it's a French word." She immediately said, "Yes! . . . Tell me." I then said, "In LIEU." She replied, "Yup!" and then went on to say, "Trouble is you know too much about words, because anybody else would just go along with (chuckles) . . ." seemingly implying that others would not engage her actively in response to her having said that that (view) was not the word she wanted to use.

So in these two cases we see how the beginning sound of a word can be correct but the rest of the word incorrect (with Mr. K) and how the opposite can also be true in the case of Dr. M. In both cases, we see that AD has affected their ability to find the correct word, but in both cases we see how it is possible to learn from these and understand that there may exist a kind of logic behind the errors. Knowing this can help us in facilitating communication, a topic I take up in a subsequent chapter.

Another of the defining characteristics of dementia in general and a result of brain injury due to AD is difficulty with what is loosely called *executive function*. The term *executive function* refers to a number of aspects of thinking, such as decision-making, planning ahead, hypothetical thinking, problem solving, initiating action, inhibiting action, self-monitoring, concept formation, attention, and reasoning (Baudic et al., 2006; McKhann et al., 2011). On standard neuropsychological tests, people with very mild AD show decrements in these abilities. Although such findings have emerged from studies such as that by Baudic and colleagues, it is also clear that some people in the moderate to severe stage of AD are still able to show intact executive functioning in natural social situations. So, as I noted in Chapter 1, there can be clear differences in what people with AD or another type of dementia accomplish in clinical testing situations compared with everyday life situations. It is very important for care partners to realize this and not make the person diagnosed a prisoner of negative stereotypes that emerge often from testing situations. For example, in the case of Dr. M (Sabat, 2001), the neuropsychologist's report about her included decrements in memory, abstraction, concept formation, and word finding that were consistent with a diagnosis of probable AD. In addition, she could no longer sign her name, use eating utensils, or dress herself (all forms of apraxia). Of interest here, however, is her executive function ability. According to standard neuropsychological tests, she showed decrements in concept formation and abstraction. Yet, in everyday life, she revealed clear ability to think abstractly and engage in hypothetical, conceptual thought, including insight into her own sad, depressed, and frustrated state of mind at the time. In a conversation with her (Sabat, 2001, p. 77) about my wanting to focus her attention on abilities that she had that were still intact, I said,

"From my point of view, I would want to work on not focusing solely, not focusing only, on what doesn't work—not to say everything is roses, and not to say that everything is garbage."

She replied, "That's nicely said."

I continued, "Thank you. But it's easy to say that everything is garbage because,"

She then interrupted me and said, "No, no, no, no. Oh yes, I do! You're right. I, I, treating things that they are garbage." To which I replied, "Because there are some things that are important to you and you can't do them, and so (you feel as if) everything is terrible . . ."

To which she responded, "Well, I tell you, I think, I'm, uh, causing that myself."

Here, Dr. M, diagnosed in the moderate to severe stage of probable AD, was able to engage in a level of honest, self-examination and gained insight into her own responsibility for feeling as she was feeling. There are many people deemed healthy who have great difficulty in achieving this level of insight into their own condition, thereby taking responsibility in important ways for their state of being. All of which is to say that executive function may appear to be dysfunctional in a variety of ways as seen in clinical testing situations, but it may be better in everyday life situations in some people diagnosed with AD or another type of dementia.

A very important ability that can have a tremendous effect on our everyday experience is called *selective attention*. Selective attention involves a number of different functions. Three such functions are (1) filtering out what we deem to be extraneous sights and sounds, (2) dividing our attention so as to do two things at once, and (3) processing incoming information quickly and efficiently. Here, I address each of these in order.

Ordinarily, we are bombarded with sights, sounds, smells, bodily sensations, and the like, and if we experienced all of them equally in every waking moment, we would be overwhelmed because no one of them would be standing out any more than any other and we would experience

tremendous confusion. For example, when sitting in a restaurant and having a conversation with a person across the
table, we have to "filter out" the sounds of other people's
voices, music in the background, movements of servers, the
feeling of our backs touching the back of the chair on which
we are sitting, the feeling of eating utensils in our hands,
and more. In order to accomplish this "filtering out," we
use brain systems that allow us to inhibit our awareness of
everything else going on around us, and the voice of our
interlocutor then stands out. Some of us might, because of
the effort involved in all this, choose to go to a quieter restaurant instead. But the world is not a restaurant, and sometimes we have no choice but to work hard to filter out all
that is insignificant to us at the moment.

People with probable AD and other types of dementia
have increasing difficulty in accomplishing this goal of filtering out "background noise," even though they want to
do so. This is because the disease has damaged brain systems that are important to this process. The example of Dr. B
(Sabat, 2001) at the adult day center is instructive. Dr. B and
I were having a good conversation in the rather peaceful
atmosphere of the staff office at the center when the level
of activity suddenly increased dramatically. People were
coming into and leaving the office, the phones were ringing
and were being answered by staff members who were then
talking with the callers, and although I was not having any
difficulty filtering out (inhibiting my awareness of) all those
extraneous sights and sounds, Dr. B was having quite a lot of
difficulty. As a result, he said, "Can we go somewhere else?
There are too many stimuli in here." This was a very cogent
observation and proper request, considering he was not able
to tune out, as it were, the office noise. Many months later,
the brain damage due to the disease worsened and we were
in the same situation in the same office. Instead of simply
asking to go elsewhere, Dr. B shut his eyes, covered his ears

with his hands (to block out the sounds), and began to cry. He was feeling overwhelmed by all the sensory stimuli and felt, it seemed, helpless and frustrated.

In this example, we can appreciate how brain damage can disrupt the abilities we use and take for granted every day. Dr. B was unable to inhibit, block out, the incoming sensations that he did not want to be dominating his experience. If we can understand his predicament and its roots in brain dysfunction, we can begin to appreciate what might be called a "dementia friendly" environment in which there is an absence of extraneous noises. A Las Vegas casino would not be "dementia friendly."

The second ability that is aided by intact brain mechanisms of selective attention is the ability to do two things at once, something that requires that we divide our attention but continuing to attend to two tasks simultaneously. There are limits to what otherwise healthy people can do when it comes to multitasking. For example, in recent years, it has become apparent that writing and sending text messages while driving a car can have deadly results. On the other hand, ironing a shirt while watching television is eminently feasible. People with AD, however, begin to lose this ability to divide their attention between two tasks as a result of the brain damage that the disease produces. As a result, the performance of one of the tasks, or both, will be negatively affected. One reason for this is that the person with AD may have difficulty inhibiting his or her awareness of and/or reactions to irrelevant features of the environment that may be present (Slavin et al., 2002).

As a result, the third ability involved with selective attention, the speed with which the person diagnosed can do all sorts of tasks, even the most familiar of tasks, will be slower than in healthier days. This reality due to brain injury and the diagnosed person's reaction to it are important for care partners to know for reasons that I explore in a subsequent chapter.

*Are there medications that can be of value to people
with Alzheimer's disease?*

To date, the US Food and Drug Administration has approved
five medications for use regarding symptoms of AD. The
drug names and brand names (in parentheses) are as follows: donepezil (Aricept), galantamine (Razadyne), memantine (Namenda), rivastigmine (Exelon), and a combination of
donepezil and memantine (Namzarac).

How do these drugs work?

These drugs work at the level of the synapses, or spaces, between
neurons in the brain. Normally, neurons transmit signals to one
another via chemicals (neurotransmitters) that are released from
the terminals of one neuron and that stimulate the next neurons
so that the process can continue. One of the important chemical
transmitters is acetylcholine (Ach). When it is released into the
synapse and stimulates the next neuron, it is then broken down
by another chemical, acetylcholinesterase (AchE), and reab-
sorbed by the terminals of the first neuron. This process readies
the synapse for another transmission—another release of Ach.
AD ultimately destroys neurons at the synapses and kills neurons
entirely, thereby disrupting the flow of information in the brain.

In order to try to make the Ach work longer in the synapses,
thereby enhancing communication between neurons, drugs
such as donepezil (Aricept), rivastigmine (Exelon), and galantamine (Razadyne) are used. These drugs are called cholines-
terase inhibitors. They inhibit AchE so that Ach in the synapses
stays there longer than usual.

The drug memantine (Namenda) is used to regulate the
activity of another important neurotransmitter, glutamate. In
AD, an excess of glutamate can be released from damaged neurons, and this can speed up damage to the cells. Memantine
partially blocks the effect of glutamate on cells, preventing cal-
cium from entering the cells and creating unwanted damage.

Do the drugs help everyone?

No. The effectiveness of such drugs varies among people. They help some to different degrees for varying lengths of time as AD progresses, but for other people they do not seem to help a great deal at all, even though they help somewhat. Some drugs may work better for some people, whereas other drugs may work better for other people.

Why is this the case?

One important reason for this is that the researchers who conduct clinical trials to determine whether or not a drug is efficacious most often use "inferential statistics" to analyze the data from two groups of people: the placebo group and the experimental group. The experimental group is given the drug in question and is followed for months at a time and given standard neuropsychological tests at the beginning of the study, during the study, and after the study ends. The placebo group receives no drug, is given a sugar pill or some such, but is given the same tests at the same times as are given to the experimental group. The groups are matched for age, education, and diagnosis of AD. Once the data are collected, they are analyzed using statistical methods that compare the two groups' results, often the averages of the groups on the tests they were given throughout the trial. If the group data from those taking the drug are statistically better than those of the placebo group, the drug is deemed efficacious.

The problem here is that the results of the group do not necessarily apply to each and every individual in the group. So even in the clinical trial, the drug may not have worked for some people, but this fact is obscured because "on the average" the group with the drug did better than did the placebo group.

This means that Aricept, or any other drug, may be helpful for some people but not for others, so if your loved one is not responding to one or another drug, there is no reason to despair for a couple of reasons. One is that the nature of drug efficacy trials and the methods of analysis employed by researchers never promised that a particular efficacious drug will actually work for everyone. A second reason not to despair is that drugs are not the only answer, as will be discussed in subsequent chapters, and their effects are generally modest anyway.

What about using drugs to treat BPSD (so-called behavioral and psychological symptoms of dementia)?

Ballard and Hulford (2006) provide an excellent, although brief, examination of drugs such as Haldol, risperidone, olanzapine, and others as they are used to treat delusions, hallucinations, anxiety, agitation, apathy, and hypomania. They recommend the following:

1. In most cases, it is preferable to use nonpharmacological treatments.
2. With regard to severe symptoms (those that put people at risk), drugs can contribute to management, but benefits have to be weighed against the adverse effects.
3. Pharmacological treatment needs to be reviewed often and stopped if ineffective or following relief of symptoms.

These recommendations are further supported by research indicating that only 10 percent of psychotropic drug use in people diagnosed with dementia was fully appropriate (van der Spek et al., 2016).

We have thus far explored a number of different alterations in the ability of the person diagnosed with AD and noted that they result from brain damage produced by the disease. We have also discussed what drug treatments can entail. If we were to end our discussion of what "everyone needs to know" about AD and other types of dementia here, we would be missing out on a great deal of information that has the potential to be of significant help to those diagnosed as well as to their care partners. One source of information that is very important to learn about and from is the *subjective experience* of the person diagnosed. This is the topic of Chapter 3.

3

ALZHEIMER'S DISEASE

THE SUBJECTIVE EXPERIENCE

The biomedical approach to Alzheimer's disease (AD) and dementia in general during most of the 20th century limited the general public's knowledge about AD primarily to what was wrong with people, and those diagnosed were often described in the mass media as "empty shells." Thus, AD in particular and dementia in general inspired and continue to inspire great fear. In the mass media, dementia has been portrayed as leaving the body healthy while taking away the mind, oddly ignoring the fact that the brain is part of the body and that AD and other causes of dementia damage the brain. The often striking, serious dysfunctions in certain aspects of thinking and perception, as discussed in Chapter 2, were emphasized most frequently, and it was assumed tacitly that that was all there was to know about AD, save for which medications to use to deal with the various "signs and symptoms," such as depression, anxiety, combativeness, and irrational hostility.

In the late 1980s and the 1990s, however, a new perspective appeared in the nonmedical professional literature, and an important part of that perspective is captured in an insightful observation made by the late, renowned neurologist, Oliver Sacks: It is one thing to know about the disease a person has but quite another to know about the person the disease has. What is it like to have AD and other dementias from the perspective of the person diagnosed? Does that person have a perspective worth taking seriously at all? Could he or she communicate about what life is like with dementia? What could others do that a person diagnosed would find helpful and that might make moments and days better than they otherwise might be? What is especially saddening to him or her? Does he or she feel good about anything and, if so, what? Could he or she feel happiness or fulfillment at all? Could he or she enjoy the company of friends and even make new friends? The list can go on, but the important point here is that the person with AD was essentially voiceless in all this, and so our understanding regarding the person diagnosed was sorely lacking.

It seemed that few, if any, medical professionals were exploring these and related questions, and if any did, they were not publishing the answers either in professional journals or in mass media outlets; even to this day, such articles are rare indeed. Instead, what we saw were articles by professional writers such as Eleanor Cooney's (2001) "Death in Slow Motion" about her mother who was diagnosed with AD and Jonathan Franzen's (2001) "My Father's Brain: What Alzheimer's Takes Away." These articles by accomplished well-known authors, as well as recent similar articles, highlight everything that is amiss, sad, annoying, and negatively challenging about the person diagnosed who, tellingly, has very little voice in these articles. There were, however, moments in both stories that could have raised an eyebrow even on the face of a person who was not educated about the remaining strengths of people with AD. I shall provide one example from Franzen's article.

In a remarkably telling narrative, Franzen (2001) describes taking his father, Earl, from the nursing home where the latter resided to the family home for Thanksgiving dinner. There was no expression of delight on his father's face upon entering the family home—his home for so long—because, as Franzen wrote, "by then, a change of venue no more impressed my father than it does a 1-year old" (p. 89). Beyond assuming *quite incorrectly* that 1-year-old children cannot discriminate a change of venue (they actually can, according to Hayne, Boniface, and Barr (2000), Barr and Hayne (2000), and other researchers), Franzen's remarkably negative stereotypic assumption about his father was itself challenged decisively by his own report about what his father said upon being brought back to the nursing home after dinner. As they sat in the car outside the nursing home, Franzen reported the following: " 'Better not to leave,' he told me in a strong voice, 'than to have to come back' " (p. 89). Franzen opined that in saying this, his father "was requesting that he be spared the pain of being dragged back toward consciousness and memory" (p. 89). Although Franzen could have meant a number of things here, I have a rather specific interpretation of what his father, Earl, was saying:

1. Being in his cherished family home for the few hours for Thanksgiving dinner was, sadly, only a painful tease because he could not remain living there as he wished.
2. Rather than being reminded of all he no longer had but still wished for, such as living in his own home, he felt that it would be "better not to leave" the nursing home at all because "to have to come back" to the nursing home after having been at home for a few hours is even more painful than living in the nursing home each and every day.
3. He knows he must live in the nursing home. He feels stuck, helpless, sad, and exiled. Being at home for a short while reminded him in painful ways of how much he had lost and he would prefer not to have that reminder.

Indeed, Earl Franzen surely was *deeply impressed by a change of venue*, although in far more significantly nuanced ways than would be true of a 1-year old. And this reaction is but one aspect of the tremendously important subject of this chapter, the subjective experience of the person diagnosed—a subject essentially ignored for decades but of signal importance to anyone who has an interest in enhancing the quality of life of people diagnosed and that of their care partners.

Why is it important to understand "the person the disease has" and how can we do so?

If we want to know how best to help another person, diagnosed with dementia or not, we need to understand that person, understand what matters most to him or her, what the person finds enlivening, what the person finds painful. What are the person's hopes and wishes? How, if at all, can they be realized? We need to have a sympathetic and, if possible, empathetic understanding of the other person. In order to achieve this level of understanding, we must assume that it is possible to do so in the first place. We must assume that we can communicate and be with the person diagnosed in ways that earn trust and respect and create an intimate understanding. In order to earn trust and respect, however, first we must learn to *give* trust and respect to the person diagnosed. Part of that process is to be open to how the person diagnosed feels and what he or she thinks and to work cooperatively with the person so as to achieve clear communication. We have to make it clear through our own words and actions that we want to listen, to understand, to help, and to comfort, and we have to believe that in so doing, the person diagnosed will understand and appreciate the intention, at the very least.

An illustration of this is my interaction with Mr. R, a retired executive and veteran of World War II who had been diagnosed with AD and who attended an adult day center twice a week. When I first encountered him, he was standing in the day center hallway, and I greeted him warmly. He responded with rapid, agitated speech, the meaning of which I did not understand save for the fact that he was uttering many words that were, in and of themselves, coherent. His face was full of frowns, and his posture and movements reflected great urgency, shaking his head while he spoke. He spoke for approximately 3 minutes and I listened, recognizing that he seemed extremely upset, although I did not know why. At one point, he paused for a moment and I asked him, "Do you feel like crying?" His eyes widened and he spoke the first sentence that was completely

coherent to me: "You're damn right I do!" Clearly, he understood my question. But why was he so upset, so agitated?

He had spent virtually every day of the past 3 years with his
wife, whom he loved dearly. Now, however, she was unable to
take him with her on the various errands she needed to complete, so she enrolled him in the social program at the day center and this was his first day. He could not recall why he was
there even though his wife had explained it to him numerous
times. He was clearly aware of his diagnosis and now seemed
fearful that his wife was having an affair. After all, his wife was
a healthy, intelligent, attractive woman who he thought was
the most beautiful woman in the world. He knew that he was
unable to do a host of things that he once did easily, so perhaps it was reasonable, from the point of view of a person who
is extremely vulnerable emotionally and feeling as if he were
burdensome to her, to fear that his wife might want the company of a man with whom she could share her life in a more
fulfilling way than she could with him. No matter how unrea-
sonable or irrational that may have appeared even to his wife,
it was the reality he was experiencing and that reality was, to
him, very, very real and very, very scary.

I had to take his point of view seriously, no matter how much
I might have thought, and confirmed later, that it was inaccu-
rate. So in trying to reassure him, I had to be with him first and
not dismiss his point of view as a "delusional" symptom of
AD. I spent hours with him during the following weeks and
months, talking with him, trying to learn about him. I learned
that he was, indeed, a veteran of World War II—that he was, in
his words, "The Top Guy," which, I learned, referred to the fact
that he was a pilot of a combat aircraft. Although he was unable
to tell me the day of the week, the season, the present location,
and had great difficulty expressing himself verbally, he was
very positively responsive to those who expressed interest in
him and tried to connect with him in an authentic way. He came
to call me "good friend" and would frequently state "You're a
good friend, God bless you" to me because he never recalled

my name. The overarching point here is that he understood and remembered my good intentions toward him and recognized me from week to week. Pointing to me, he once commented to one of the student interns, "That man is still trying to get in. He wants in, but I can't tell many others. He's trying, though, God bless him." He understood, therefore, that I was trying to "get in"—to understand—his thoughts and feelings.

So the first step in trying to understand what life is like for the person with dementia is to connect with him or her on an open, honest, level and to take seriously what the person says, commiserating with his or her fears or anxieties, extending words of comfort and concern. No matter the person's lack of "orientation to time and place," he or she seems to be able to understand good intentions when they are displayed in the actions of another person.

What is it like to experience the process of being diagnosed with Alzheimer's disease?

Lisa Snyder, former Director of Quality of Life Programs, ran support groups for people with AD at the Shiley–Marcos Alzheimer's Disease Research Center at the University of California, San Diego for 27 years, and connected deeply with people diagnosed. In her especially revealing, important book, *Speaking Our Minds: What It's Like to Have Alzheimer's*, Snyder (2009) encouraged people diagnosed with AD to speak about their experiences, some of which involved the health care professions. Two of the seven people whose stories are presented in the book, Bea and Betty, related their experiences with medical professionals. Bea said of the neurologist who interviewed her,

> He was very indifferent and said it was just going to get worse. ... If he had just shown a little compassion. He was there to diagnose my problem, but he wasn't there to understand my feelings. He had no feelings for me whatsoever. I've hated him ever since. Health care professionals need to be compassionate. (p. 19)

Betty, a former faculty member at San Diego State University and a retired social worker, made the following comment about the health care professionals she encountered during the process of being diagnosed:

> They're busy wanting to climb up to the next rung on the ladder. That's very human. I don't blame them. But they don't really accept the significance of the illness for people. They know the diagnosis, but they don't take time to find out what it truly means for that person. This casualness with which professionals deal with Alzheimer's is so painful to see. . . . A person with Alzheimer's disease is many more things than just their diagnosis. Each person is a whole human being. . . . You have to really be willing to be present with the person who has Alzheimer's. But there are some people who don't want to learn, and it's the looking down on and being demeaning of people with Alzheimer's that is hard to watch. (pp. 123–124)

Clearly, it is incorrect to assume that interactions of this type occur in each and every situation between health care professionals and their patients, but it surely was true in these cases, as it was in the case of Dr. B, whose internist commented that "treating a person with Alzheimer's is like doing veterinary medicine." There are many health care professionals who do not think this way at all, but it is clear from the experiences of many people diagnosed that we still have much room for improvement in the way people with AD are treated.

Another person with whom Snyder worked was Bill, who discussed a great deal about his experience of AD, including being diagnosed (Snyder, 2009):

> At age 54, it seemed like I was labeled incompetent after a lifetime of proficiency. The psychologist who tested me said that I would find it increasingly arduous to work, or

even drive a car. I was devastated. After the diagnosis, I remember walking out of the clinic and into a fresh San Diego night feeling like a very hopeless and broken man. The next morning, the neurologist apologized for the psychologist's lack of tact. . . . The scariest time in this whole process was that first diagnosis. I wondered if there was anything for me to live for. It was an awful time. (p. 41)

What is it like for a person to have Alzheimer's disease?

If you have met one person with AD, you have met one person with AD. There is no "one size fits all" when it comes to understanding how people experience and react to the losses they incur due to the disease. In many cases, the reaction depends on the value the person placed on particular aspects of life in decades before the diagnosis, how he or she has dealt with adversity in the past, and what the person's style of being happens to be. Although I discuss particular people herein, I am not at all implying that all people with AD are precisely like the ones whom I discuss. Just the same, there can be valuable lessons to learn from each person.

For example, Dr. B, a retired professor, was in the moderate to severe stage of AD according to standard tests. For most of his adult life, he was an avid reader and loved to learn. But now, he was having great difficulty reading, and this, combined with his difficulty in speaking in erudite English (another of his abilities in the past), led him to describe his difficulty in reading as follows (Sabat, 2001):

I think I was getting some good, um, also the Alzheimer's is, uh, tears me apart on it. It comes to the point of how to read for me . . . it doesn't work for me and um, I fell [he meant "felt"] a lot of antagonize to myself. (p. 36)

For a time, though, he was able to read (the effects can vary from moment to moment), but then the problems surfaced and he wondered about his ability: *"Is it still mine?"* So he was angry with himself and sad and frustrated because he could not do something that was so much a part of his life for so long—something that he, just as is the case with most of us, took for granted until it was no longer the simple task it had been for so many years. And so now he grieved.

The same Dr. B said the following when I asked him what he thinks of when I say the word "Alzheimer's" (Sabat, 2001):

> Um, mad as hell ... constantly on my mind ... everything that dominates me now is Alzheimer's. ... I think about the delumision [diminution], you know, of what I've been able to do, and what I may never do. ... I know prominently that I have Alzheimer's and I can't, can't stop it ... something's knocked me down and I can't do anything about it. (p. 30)

Here, he describes a very understandable feeling of sadness, frustration, and helplessness in that he cannot do anything to stop the diminution of what he was once able to do. Beyond that, he is aware that the disease may mean that in the future he will not be able to do things he had once planned.

Among the most important points to be understood about Dr. B is that he is able to reflect accurately on what AD means to him and what it will mean for him and for his family. His diagnosis of AD in the moderate to severe stages did not prevent him from having a very appropriate, cogent reaction to its effects. This means that AD can affect *some* aspects of thinking but not all aspects. He can still evaluate the meaning of the disease and its effects, and this is something he carries with him each day, even though he may not recall which day of the week it happens to be or what county he is in, perform rudimentary numerical calculations, or dress himself. In order to know all this, one would have to have engaged Dr. B in an open, honest way, earned his trust, and worked to understand what he was trying to convey, even though he mispronounced words occasionally and did not always speak in complete, syntactically correct, sentences.

Another person who reflected clearly on her experience of AD was Dr. M, a retired professor whom I mentioned briefly in Chapter 2 and whose life was marked by her having been, in the words of her husband, "fiercely independent." Her powerful intellect was matched by her graceful, exceptionally sophisticated, use of the English language. She agreed wholeheartedly when I stated that for her, words were like a musical instrument; she had a lifelong love of graceful, even poetic, expression. So it was quite natural that she would say, "You know what? Because I don't speak like I used to be, it seems to me that I don't have any good way of speaking," and she agreed strongly when I asked if she was dissatisfied with that and further stated that as a result, "I'm being angry with myself" (Sabat, 2001, p. 70). She had always been very good with people, very witty and an excellent conversationalist, but the effects of AD led her to say, "Among the may [many] important things, I can't talk to people" and "these are most of the moments in my life now and I don't want that" (p. 75). So of course she was saddened and wanting very much to regain her former skills. She was so deeply distressed by her losses that when I asked her what she thought she did well, she could not give me one example because "the most things that I'm that's . . . that I, uh, keep my eye on or notice is not for the best" (p. 76). In the presence of such a person, one cannot but feel great compassion and sympathize with the grief that she experienced. Furthermore, one feels almost compelled to try to help her find and acknowledge all the good qualities that she still possesses in abundance rather than allow her to drown in a sea of solitary frustration and grief.

Not everyone is as open about their emotional reactions as were Dr. B and Dr. M. Indeed, there are people who rarely, if ever, express their emotions so openly. For example, Gen. U, a retired career army officer who landed in Normandy at Omaha

Beach on D-Day, was diagnosed with dementia, though not of the Alzheimer's type. Although he did say to his wife on one occasion, "I know you never thought our life together would come to this" in connection with his diagnosis, he rarely expressed anger or frustration. In one of the more than 1,200 e-mail letters that his wife and I exchanged over a period of 3 years about how she could improve her understanding of his condition and thereby improve her ability to provide loving support for him, she asked, "Wouldn't you be angry if you couldn't remember things that you knew you should remember? My husband doesn't seem to show any kind of reaction at all." I responded,

> Well, perhaps you and I would be angry and show it, but neither of us is your husband. You know more about him than I do, so perhaps you can think about this: How has he typically handled adversity in all the decades you have known him?

This question prompted her to reflect on her husband in connection with his way of expressing himself under dire conditions, and she realized that he never showed any outward reactions—that he was always on an even keel in the face of adversity. And so in this situation, he was acting very much as he always did in the past (Sabat, 2011).

Symptoms of disease or reactions to losses?

The sadness and frustration expressed by Dr. B and Dr. M and the agitation and fear expressed by Mr. R should not be thought of as " signs and symptoms" of AD in the same way that fever is a symptom of malaria or red spots on the skin are a sign of measles. Rather, these feelings should be thought of as *logical, normal reactions* to the losses that dementia means. How would you feel if you were no longer able to read well or do other things that you always relished and did effortlessly, such as signing your name? Dr. M could no longer do that. Would you be delighted? Would you not care at all? You might very well be distraught and rightly so, perhaps embarrassed and angry as well. People with dementia can react in very reasonable ways to their losses, and their reactions should not be "pathologized" by making them into "symptoms of disease." An antidepressant would not necessarily change the reality of what the situation meant for Dr. B and for Dr. M. In fact, if they did not react as they did, it would be worrisome and they would then be characterized as being "blissfully unaware" of, or "in denial" about, their defects—a symptom of illness called *anosognosia*. So you see how, either way, what is a perfectly reasonable reaction to a loss, expressed or not expressed, can be made to appear as if it were a symptom of disease. Interpreting a logical reaction in this way does not give the person diagnosed credit for being able to react, and act, much as would any healthy person to the loss of an important ability or to react as he or she always has to adversity.

Other examples of the mislabeling of a person's reaction to the effects of AD are found when a person becomes angered or cries convulsively in particular situations. For instance, during clinical testing, a person with dementia might become furious and curse, cry, or even walk out of the testing room upon failing to answer what could be viewed as relatively simple questions on standard tests. The medically oriented description of this is that the person is displaying a "catastrophic reaction" or is "emotionally labile," and these are interpreted as being symptoms of dementia. Of course, we could just as easily interpret these as rather logical reactions to the horror of failing "in public" to do something that the person knows is simple and that he or she could have done easily in the past. Perhaps this failure is the "straw that breaks the camel's back" when viewed in the larger context of the person not being able to do many things that were once rather simple, even automatic. Similarly, a well-intentioned and loving spousal care partner conveyed that "whenever the nurse is going to come to the house to give my wife a bath, my wife cries convulsively and I cannot help her to calm down before the nurse arrives." He thought that her crying was symptomatic of dementia (she was diagnosed with AD) until we discussed the situation further. I suggested to him that his wife could very well (1) feel extremely uncomfortable about being naked in the presence of someone who is essentially a stranger to her; (2) feel embarrassed, and even humiliated, by the fact that she now needs someone to help her with basic personal hygiene; and (3) feel completely out of control of a number of fundamental aspects of adult life, bathing being one. The husband very solemnly said that he had never thought of it that way and that, knowing his wife as he did for so many decades, he could understand very well that she would feel that way and thus cry convulsively. Losing control over a number of everyday situations can be very distressing to persons with dementia, just as it would be to anyone otherwise deemed healthy.

Another example is clearly stated by Dr. B, who always enjoyed taking healthy walks before the onset of AD. At the day center, he was frustrated because he was not allowed to go for a walk outside without someone with him. Although this was an understandable prohibition from the standpoint of the day center's liability, from Dr. B's point of view, it was quite different, as he said, "*I want very much to be independent.* Right now, I can't go out without anybody else . . . and it irritates me. . . . I find I want to get away from the lock-step." He felt rather closed in by the day center's regulations. It is quite important to have such conversations in which people are allowed to express their desires and frustrations and feel understood. After all, not being able to go for a walk by himself was not the only way in which Dr. B had lost a measure of the independence he experienced for decades of adult life, and it is vital for care partners to be aware of and understanding about such a serious loss so as, at the very least, to commiserate with the person diagnosed.

One must also consider the person who lives in a nursing home, who cannot leave, who must eat at a particular time whether or not he or she is hungry, who has lost the ability to make a host of independent choices in life, and who may not recall the last time a loved one visited. This person can feel imprisoned and alone and might break down and cry convulsively out of sheer loneliness and frustration. Giving this person drugs to "tranquilize" him or her will not remove the reasons for deep distress and loneliness, which are quite reasonable feelings under the circumstances.

How can attention problems due to dementia affect a person's experience?

Another very important aspect of the subjective experience of AD is found in what Dr. B said quite directly: "Things get jumbled and Alzheimer's gives me fragments." That is, due to problems with retrieving information about recent events via recall and the wavering of his attention, he believes that he does not always have the "whole picture" of situations as they transpire. He has, instead, small pieces, or fragments, of what is happening or has happened. This is especially true if events around him are happening at a rapid pace and he cannot process them all as quickly and as efficiently as he did before AD or if he is experiencing heightened anxiety. Just the same, however, it is very important to realize that he can reflect so accurately on his experience. That AD gives him fragments is true, but it is also true that he understands this entirely and not in a fragmented way at all. Thus, he can know clearly that his experience of external events can be fragmented. If people around him understand this, they can work with him so that he can begin to understand the "whole picture."

This was exactly the case in one of my early conversations with Dr. B in which he wanted his wife and me to meet and for her to provide information that would be useful to "The Project," as he referred to our work together. Apparently, during the previous weekend, he was insisting to his wife that she speak to me and she kept telling him that she would do so when I contacted her to arrange a meeting, as per our agreement. In his urgency about all this, he was, unfortunately, not assimilating that "fragment" and kept insisting to her that she and I speak, and she kept repeating to him that she would do so when I contacted her. He felt that something was, as he said, "eroshing in our life"—that there was some erosion in his marriage, as she was becoming exasperated with him. It took approximately 15 minutes of back-and-forth discussion about this for me to fill in the piece he was missing and to assure him that I would contact her. He then finally said, "All right. If it will be, that was pushing too much." Here, he showed a clear, accurate insight into the fact that he had been insisting too much and not hearing what his wife was saying to him. In order for him to come to this realization, however, I had to listen to him patiently and carefully, recognize and honor the great emotion that was involved in his feeling of urgency that his wife and I meet and his additional fear that there was a problem with his marriage, and understand that he was missing the important "fragment" of what his wife was telling him. Then, I had to assure him repeatedly that, as far as I could tell, his marriage was not eroding.

Simultaneously, Dr. B can have thoughts, lose track of them, wait a while, and they come back to him. If he is distracted in the middle of a conversation, it would be most helpful not to interrupt him with a statement or a question when he is pausing to retrieve the thread of the conversation. Instead, it would be most helpful to remain silent, allowing him to think without distraction. Extended silence in the middle of a conversation is often uncomfortable for many people, but this is one very important adaptation that is critical to make for the sake of the person diagnosed. There are times in the middle of conversations with people who have AD that I have remained silent for 30 seconds or more (try measuring it), allowing my interlocutor time to retrieve a thought without being distracted by something I might say. We can appreciate this in the following interchange between Dr. B and me (Sabat, 2001, p. 39):

> DR. B: When I leave something with hiatus, I think maybe I get, I wouldn't say disturbed, but it, it it screws up the rhythm.
>
> SRS: Oh, so if you're in the middle of thinking about something,
>
> DR. B: Uh huh
>
> SRS: And you get distracted,
>
> DR. B: Yeah
>
> SRS: Then you lose what you wanted to say?
>
> DR. B: Yeah, but um, I can, uh wait for a little while
>
> SRS: Um-hum
>
> DR. B: And uh, I get rejuvenation, and uh, up it comes.

Thus, we have to allow the person with AD extra time to formulate and then retrieve thoughts and words without interruption because even saying, "What did you want to say?" is, itself, just another distraction. Distractions, however, can come in very different, unanticipated, forms.

Dr. M's ability to focus her attention on one thing completely was compromised by AD as well, and as a result, she could lose track of what it was she wanted to say even in the middle of speaking a sentence. One blatant example occurred when she was speaking to me and interrupted herself and said, "I can't say it now, but it, it is, let me think and not look at you . . . I have been looking at you all the time because you look like somebody I know" (Sabat, 2001, p. 71). In the middle of saying something to me, it occurred to her that I looked like someone she knows and she lost track of what she was trying to say initially because she was then trying to think of the identity of the person of whom I reminded her. It turned out that it was one of her sons who bore a resemblance to me. The point of this example is to alert care partners that the focused attention of a person with AD or another type of dementia can be interrupted by another thought and that thought can serve to disrupt what the person is saying because now there are two competing thoughts occurring simultaneously. In order to know if this is what is happening, there has to be an open, trusting relationship in place so that the person with AD is assured that he or she will not be judged as being "defective" when such things happen. Many of us experience having second and third thoughts occur to us as we are speaking to another person, but we are able to inhibit our attention to those other thoughts and continue saying what we set out to say. One problem that occurs with dementia is that the person may not be able to inhibit those other competing thoughts and, thus, loses track of what he or she is saying at the moment.

Can a person with Alzheimer's disease experience happiness?

It may sound obvious, but it is important to state nonetheless, given the pervasive negative stereotypes about AD: People with AD or any form of dementia are people first. As is true for people without a diagnosis of dementia, people with AD can be sad and frustrated about some aspects of their lives and simultaneously happy about others. For example, not everything was saddening to Dr. B. When I asked him what made him happy, he replied, "Well, number one is the light of my life [his wife of many decades, to whom he frequently referred that way when he did not use her first name]. That's one thing. Um, and then, uh, the rest of my life is the, uh, my children, about three or four. . . . So the world to me still lives." He was always tremendously devoted to and involved with his family, and that did not change with AD and neither did many of his other admirable attributes.

As is true for most of us, there were things about which he was anxious and needed some encouragement from others, such as his wife, in order to cope effectively. For example, he conveyed to me that "I still need bucking up and uh, I think my wife prods me every so often and she's right . . ."

in connection with some anxiety he felt about taking a long plane ride across the country to visit a sick, older relative. He always disliked flying, and AD did not change that feeling. He not only needed encouragement, but he also needed to be able to talk about how he felt about things on a day-to-day basis: "I sure do ... really glad, you know, you let me ventilate." In these two domains—the need for gentle encouragement and the need to be able to "ventilate" or talk about how one is feeling—we see this person with AD as being no different from many people without a diagnosis. Many of us can relate to such needs quite easily. How encouragement is given and how the space for conversation and "ventilation" is created may be different from person to person, but the need for and benefit of both are as clear in the case of some people with dementia as in the case of some people without a diagnosis.

As with Dr. B, Dr. M also experienced happiness, perhaps delight, even though she had her moments of despair and frustration. One moment of delight occurred at the end of one of our hour-long conversations that began with her saying that she could not think of anything about which she felt good. We wound up discussing a task that had been awaiting her attention for quite some time that involved organizing some of her professional papers for a university library that expressed an interest in them and how it was important for her not to procrastinate about that task. She commented, "This was a good session, don't you think?" and continued, "Um, I'm not the fir, the first, the real person that came out when you, before when you ... came on this, uh, day, is different." I took this to mean something akin to "I'm not the same person as the one who greeted you when you first came today." She went on to say, in a very positive, thoughtful way, "I, I, I need to find for myself what are the real important things in uh, one person's life." Although at the outset of this conversation, Dr. M could not think of anything that she did well and was mired in the negative thoughts about her condition, by the end of the conversation, she had identified a project that was important for her to see through to its logical end and to identify what is really important in her life and to attempt to achieve some positive goals. Thus, she felt as if she were a different person from the one who greeted me upon my arrival at her home that day. The conversation we had was therapeutic for her, for she, too, "ventilated" about her feelings.

In time, I became the co-leader of Dr. M's support group, and when we met for our regular conversations, we often discussed the dynamics of the previous support group meeting a week earlier. Her recollection of the meetings was remarkably accurate in many ways. After one long conversation in which we discussed a situation that occurred at the previous meeting during which she observed a reaction of one of the group members to something she said, she said with utter delight, "It seems to me, uh, that that's int, interesting and I just love going through things like that" (Sabat, 2001, p. 188). This kind of discussion was perfectly in line with her long-standing proclivities, for after she retired from her university faculty position, she earned a master's degree in social work, seeking to become a psychotherapist. Unfortunately, soon thereafter, her memory problems began and she was unable to realize that goal.

Still another example of Dr. M experiencing delight occurred during a conversation in which she used gestures to communicate when she could not find the words she wanted to use. She often expressed her despair over not being able to speak beautifully as she did in the past. On some of these occasions, I tried to convey to her that she was still communicating well and that it is quite possible to communicate clearly without using any words at all, for the famous mime, Marcel Marceau, was quite successful at doing just that for decades in his professional life to the delight of audiences throughout the world. In one subsequent conversation, Dr. M could not find the word she wanted to use on two different occasions, and on each occasion, she used a gesture to convey her thought to me and I understood clearly what she was trying to convey each time. On the second occasion of my having shown that I understood her, she said, "Exactly, who needs words!!!!" and she laughed heartily. I then pointed out that she accomplished the task of communicating clearly twice by using gestures. I said, "You made your point." To which she replied, "I made *your* point," thereby revealing a very highly developed sense of wit in conveying her understanding that she just displayed exactly what I was trying to communicate to her in the first place. She was clearly amused and delighted and evinced what could be described as a kind of joy of being free—in the realization that she did not have to possess her former command and élan in the use of words in order to communicate what was important to her. So she felt free, in a way, of the limitation she experienced due to word-finding and pronunciation problems.

Do people with Alzheimer's disease or another type of dementia need and want purpose in life? Do they have a sense of proper pride and self-respect?

Yes, they definitely do, especially if they needed and sought purpose in their lives in previous decades. For example, at the adult day center, Dr. B rarely, if ever, involved himself in the usual activities that were part of the daily program, saying, "I don't necessarily need what's in that room," referring to one of the activities at the day center. Instead, he chose to spend time with me, 2 hours per day twice a week, as part of "The Project" on which he worked with me to help me understand what it is like to have Alzheimer's. The Project was tremendously important to him because it was, as he called it, "a scientific sort of thing" and "we can get glory" from this work. He asked the director of the day center to post a sign on the hallway bulletin board indicating the days and times at which we would be meeting to work on The Project. In this way, everyone at the day center knew that he was doing this work, and in this way he differentiated himself from the rest of the group, thus giving him something of pride of place there as well as a reminder of our meeting times.

In addition to his work on The Project, Dr. B made himself available to undergraduate students in my advanced seminar in clinical neuropsychology, helping them to understand what it was like to have AD. His effect on the students was clear in a letter I received from one of them, Heather Markey, upon learning of Dr. B's death:

"He was a wonderful man who taught us all so much. … No other person and no book could have taught me as much as Dr. B did. … [His] greatest quality was his ability to affect all of us who knew him. He will continue living in all of us and in all he showed us.

As someone who was a rather accomplished painter, Dr. B offered critiques of the artwork created by some of my students. His critiques of one student's work matched exactly what her professor told her. When I told him this, he said, "Yeah? And I'm a scientist, for Christ sake! [laughter]." His use of the present tense here ("I am") is extremely important and provides us with an insight into how he viewed himself. Clearly, Dr. B was no longer a practicing scientist as he was during the decades of his vocational life. Just as clearly, however, in terms of his disposition, habits of mind, and his sense of who he was, he was very much a scientist. This aspect of him deserved to be honored and respected openly. His proclivities were clear in the way he comported himself at the day center, so it would be utterly wrong to say about him, "He used to be a scientist." Indeed, Dr. B, in talking about himself and his wife of many decades, said, "Well, my wife and I are very strong academic people and, uh, so we start talking to each other, we talk to each other at a very high level right away." This plainly indicates an aspect of his disposition that he valued greatly and needed to be recognized and respected by others and now, especially, nurtured.

This idea was blatantly expressed by another day center participant, Henry, who was a retired attorney diagnosed with

AD in the moderate stage. Introducing Henry to another person, the day center director said to the other person, "This is Henry. Henry was a lawyer." Henry then interrupted and said quite assertively, "I *am* a lawyer!" Of course, Henry was still a lawyer. He had not been disbarred, after all. Although he was no longer practicing law, that fact did not change the reality of who he was in the world and in his view. His way of being, his habits of mind, clearly reflected this truth as they did for Dr. B, the scientist, and Henry's accomplishment and standing as an attorney could not and should not be dismissed or diminished simply because of his diagnosis.

Although he was warm and courteous to the other participants, Dr. B correctly viewed himself as different from them in temperament, disposition, and lifelong pursuits. He was proud of his accomplishments in life and wanted the respect he always enjoyed in his adult life. Indeed, he felt quite correctly that the people at the day center did not recognize him in this way. When I asked if he felt as if he had no status there, he said, "Oh absolutely. Absolutely! There, there, should be some hier, hierarty." He believed that his work on The Project helped to give him some status. Thus, it must be remembered by care partners of all kinds, family relations as well as professionals, that people with AD/dementia even in the moderate to severe stages can retain their pride and need for recognition of their positive qualities—just as do most of us without a diagnosis. This is especially important, though, when a person is diagnosed with AD or another type of dementia and easily can be seen primarily in terms of the diagnosis and all its related defects, which are anathema to him or her. In this situation, being seen for one's valued qualities becomes even more important than it was in past healthier days.

That Dr. B's long-standing dispositions were quite intact could be appreciated in his reaction to some of the activities that formed the daily program at the day center, especially the game Trivial Pursuit. While standing in the hall, observing the game being played inside one of the day center's rooms, I asked Dr. B what he thought of the game. He replied, "It's filler." I asked what that meant, and he said that filler is "something that doesn't mean anything—I wish I could make it break." Of course, the game required quick recall of isolated facts, and that was something that AD prevented him from doing, thus creating further frustration. He was never interested in such things, and AD did not change that about him. What he was interested in was doing something meaningful with his time, and he did not consider the games and activities at the day center to be meaningful. Thus, he was capable of appreciating the presence and absence of meaning when presented with situations such as this one.

Indeed, Dr. B needed to be able to tell others about the significant work he was doing with me, but his own word-finding problems and syntactical challenges prevented him from doing so if, for example, someone were to ask him what he was doing with his days. As a result, he needed my help to provide him with something that would speak for him, as it were. I therefore arranged for a letter of commendation to be sent to him from the Dean of Georgetown University's College of Arts and Sciences. The letter specified the many ways in which he was making a positive contribution to the education of Georgetown students and to the extant literature on AD. He was thereby recognized for his service to the community and carried a photocopy of the letter with him. It was tremendously important to him that he not be defined by AD and the dysfunctions it causes. This is perfectly in keeping with the desire most of us have to be seen for our positive, admirable attributes rather than for our foibles.

Feeling proper pride and the desire to be treated with respect and dignity requires tremendously complex brain functions, including memory, attention, emotion, and abstract thought such as the idea of fairness. Even though he could not dress himself, Dr. B was able to work to maintain his dignity and ask for reciprocity. Standard neuropsychological tests do not tap into any of these important aspects of human life and so care partners need to be aware of this fact when told that their loved one is diagnosed with AD even in the moderate to severe stages. Likewise, care partners must understand that the inability to dress oneself, use eating utensils, or sign one's name are not indicators of a lack of the kind of complex thinking that Dr. B and other people with AD have revealed.

In an experiment conducted regarding feeling a sense of purpose, Mak (2010) found that people with dementia who drew a greeting card for military personnel serving abroad or for a child who was sick reported higher levels of purpose in life than did people with dementia who made similar drawings with no specific person in mind. In this case, the purpose was significant in social terms because it connected the person with doing something for the well-being of others. In a similar way, it was very clear to Dr. B and Dr. M that the purpose of the work I was doing with them was to help others, and they eagerly cooperated with me in that pursuit. Many times, one or the other would ask me in the middle of a conversation, "Is this helping you?" This aspect of people with AD should not be surprising when one thinks about the reality of their lives. Unfortunately, it is not often that others ask a person diagnosed for his or her help. It is usually the person diagnosed who is on the receiving end of help rather than the one doing the giving. For a person in this social position, it is often a breath of fresh air to be able to help others, especially if the person with dementia spent most of his or her adult life taking delight in doing so.

Mr. K reported that his wife did nothing at home but sit or walk around aimlessly and sometimes watch television. At the day center, however, she was very active in helping others wherever and however she could, including setting the tables for the lunch meal and helping people in wheelchairs by opening doors for them. As it turned out, the reason she did nothing at home was that Mr. K did everything himself and, by his own admission, did not ask her for help because he feared that she would fail in trying to help him and he did not want her to experience failure. Although he was filled with good intentions, he unwittingly prevented her from experiencing the kind of meaning and purpose she reveled in, for she had always been a service-oriented person.

Having to make choices and take responsibility for doing things is part of normal everyday life for most adults, and it is critical for our well-being. Langer and Rodin (1976) demonstrated that people living in a nursing home benefited greatly when they were able to make choices and take responsibility in connection with matters of daily life. In one group, residents were given a series of choices about how to arrange furniture in their rooms, encouraged to tell staff if they wanted changes to be made, could choose plants for their rooms and had to take care of the plants themselves, and were told that there would be movies shown on two nights and to decide which showing they wanted to attend if they wanted to attend at all. In a second group, residents were not given the choice regarding arranging furniture, were given a plant (no choice as to which plant to take) and told that the staff would water the plants, and were told that there would be movie nights and the staff would tell them which one they were scheduled to attend. The people in the first group reported feeling happier and more active than did those in the second group. In addition, the people in the first group were rated higher by nurses (who did not know about the previously mentioned differences in choice and responsibility) on measures of alertness, interacting with others, happiness, and talking to staff members. They spent less time engaged in passive activities than did those in the second group. These effects were mirrored in connection with the health status of the groups. Thus, having the ability to make choices about relatively simple matters had profoundly positive effects psychologically and medically.

Thus, we can appreciate the insightful approach that Mrs. B revealed whenever she came to the day center to pick up Dr. B at the end of the day. They would greet each other warmly, and he would immediately say to her, "Okay, what are we doing now?" She always replied, "What would you like to do?" thus giving him the choice about what would happen next. When I asked her why she did that, she said she did not want her husband to become passive and simply do whatever she said they were going to do. Rather, she wanted him to see himself as having choices and as one whose opinion mattered to her as much as hers did to him. Thus, she sought to maintain his level of independence insofar as their activities as a couple.

The message from all this is quite clear: It is important for a person with AD to have choices and to be encouraged to assert his or her wishes wherever possible, even about seemingly simple matters, for his or her physical and mental health can be affected in a positive way as a result. This is especially important when a person has a degenerative disease.

Do still other people with Alzheimer's disease react to their losses and seek to avoid embarrassment?

Yes, but the way people do these things can vary widely depending on the person and his or her life story. For example, a kind and gracious woman, Mrs. O, was having trouble following conversations that took place at the weekly dinners that she and her husband attended with a group of friends who did not know that she had AD. During the meals, she spoke sparingly, concentrating on eating and drinking, and it is socially acceptable not to speak a great deal while eating. As soon as dessert was finished, Mrs. O immediately began clearing the table and proceeded to wash dishes and utensils. Everyone considered her actions as being wonderfully kind and considerate. Only later did Mr. O realize that this was her way of avoiding the lively conversation that ensued around the dinner table. She sought to avoid being embarrassed by her inability to respond intelligently if she were asked about her view of this or that topic of conversation, for she was unable to attend to and process the rapid comments made by the others at the table.

Mrs. D, a participant at the day center, was raised in a show business family and possessed a wonderful sense of humor. She had a high school education and was not an intellectual as were Dr. B and Dr. M. When she experienced word-finding problems, she made a joke out of them. For example, she was trying to find a particular word and could not, so she simply said, "Oh, it's that Alcazheimer's again—it's a helluva disease!" spoken with a kind of show business flair, a broad smile, raised eyebrows, all of which were anything but sad. When Dr. M experienced word-finding problems, however, she would refrain from speaking because she felt that she "couldn't talk." This was especially embarrassing to her when she attended a support group and the group leader would say, for example, "We haven't heard from you yet." This, she felt, put her on the spot, and she became insistent upon not attending the support group for a time so as to avoid such situations.

Mrs. K also attended the day center and had severe word-finding and syntactical problems in speaking sentences correctly. As a result, she was quiet most of the time. Throughout her adult life, she took great pride in her appearance and in her desire to be of help, of service, to others. As mentioned previously, she was able to help people in wheelchairs navigate through doorways if they needed help, helped organize place settings for the lunch meal, and reveled in being recognized and thanked for her concern and help. Whenever the group was about to engage in a discussion of one or another topic, she would absent herself and go for a walk in the long hallway of the building or go to another room and look through the pages of a magazine. That is, she recognized the situation as one that could lead to her being called upon to speak and so she chose to do something else instead so as to avoid the potential embarrassment.

Each of these examples reveals intact "executive function" (discussed in Chapter 1), wherein the person was able to assess the situation as being potentially harmful and engage a plan of action designed to avoid that harm. This is a type of "if

... then" hypothetical thinking wherein the person says, for example, "If I remain in this situation it will be embarrassing to me and if I don't want to be embarrassed, then I have to absent myself from this situation." So when people with AD or another type of dementia do something to avoid what could easily be embarrassing, even humiliating, their actions should be viewed as examples of adaptive behavior designed to maintain dignity and self-respect rather than their being "uncooperative" or "aloof" by leaving the small group discussion, for example. It is of utmost importance that care partners assume that there may well be, and often is, a good reason for what the diagnosed person is doing and attempt to understand that reason given the situation and the personality and needs of the individual in question.

This can be the case for situations that do not involve the person with AD trying to avoid embarrassment but, rather, the person is trying to continue to be a worthy, helpful partner to his or her spouse. Mr. F, for example, reported that his wife often "purposefully puts things in the wrong places" at home. That is, she went around the house, seemingly in the act of tidying up, but put particular objects in places where they should not be put normally. She was trying, with the best of intentions, to take care of things at home as she had always done in the past with great success while simultaneously doing a host of impressive things, including tutoring children and working in the community and winning the respect and admiration of her husband and friends. She was clearly aware that she was not being the wonderfully accomplished and helpful partner to her husband that she had been in the past decades of their marriage. Indeed, she said to her husband very poignantly, "I'm no good for you," thereby reflecting a very well-developed ability to evaluate her actions past and present as well as a sense of the deep anguish she was experiencing at present. As it was, her husband told me, "I married her for two reasons. One is that I fell head over heels in love with her. That has not changed. My feelings toward her in that regard are the same as they were before. Put it this way—I still have a crush on her." At this, he began to cry. He continued, "The other thing was I saw in her someone who would fill in what I needed. She's very forthright, she has a lot of competence; she has a lot of confidence." Mrs. F was clearly aware of the qualities that drew her husband to her and inspired his love and respect. She was just as clearly aware that she was no longer able to do all the things she used to do, hence her previously mentioned poignant comment to him. Clearly, people with AD or another type of dementia can react to their losses and feel the need to avoid embarrassment, but . . .

Can people diagnosed with Alzheimer's disease or another type of dementia experience well-being?

Yes. As I have discussed briefly already, it is possible for persons diagnosed with AD to experience happiness, delight, and seek out and enjoy having purpose in life. In addition, however, there are other forms of well-being that care partners need to be aware of and thus able to observe and appreciate in their loved ones who are diagnosed. Something of a guide to expressions of well-being was created by the late, esteemed, former Head of the Bradford Dementia Group at the University of Bradford in England, Tom Kitwood. He referred to these expressions as "indicators of relative well-being," which are areas of common ground shared by people diagnosed and those deemed healthy (Kitwood, 1998). It is important for care partners to be aware of these indicators because their presence reveals strengths possessed by persons diagnosed, and such strengths need to be acknowledged as having the value they deserve when they are displayed.

Kitwood (1998) proposed a list of 12 indicators but noted that this list is hardly exhaustive; there are many other such indicators. It is also important to understand that a person diagnosed with dementia may exhibit some or perhaps all of these indicators from time to time. There is no "threshold" number of these indicators that needs to be displayed in order for a person to have established common ground with otherwise healthy people. In other words, there is no minimum score that a person has to attain in order for him or her to be seen as being "still there." It is also important to recognize that these indicators become apparent only when there is some kind of social interaction occurring. With all this in mind, the list of indicators is as follows:

- The assertion of desire or will
- The ability to experience and express a range of emotions
- Initiation of social contact
- Affectional warmth
- Social sensitivity
- Self-respect
- Acceptance of other people with dementia
- Humor
- Creativity and self-expression
- Showing evident pleasure
- Helpfulness
- Relaxation

Mrs. H and Fr. D, participants at the adult day center, diagnosed with AD in the moderate to severe stage, provided an example of some of the previously mentioned indicators in the following dynamic social situation. I walked into a room at the center holding a small, water-soaked towel over one of my eyes due to an allergic reaction. The room was filled with participants seated at the long lunch tables because one of the daily activities was in progress. Mrs. H and Fr. D, seated across the room, seemed to notice me immediately. Both quickly arose from their chairs and walked over to me with great purpose and looks of concern on their faces. Mrs. H, who had severe word-finding problems, pointed to the towel I was holding, as if to ask, "What's wrong?" I explained why I was holding the towel over my eye, that I was okay, and thanked her and Fr. D for their concern. They nodded and returned to their chairs. Here we see the initiation of social contact, helpfulness, showing concern, and then relief (different emotions experienced and expressed), as well as the following cognitive abilities: the ability to focus attention, the ability to infer that my holding the towel over my eye signified something was wrong, the expression of concern in response, the ability to understand what I said that led to their concern being relieved, and an intact short-term memory that allowed each person to return to where they originally sat (among other empty chairs). In other words, Mrs. H and the priest both cared about me and demonstrated it clearly, revealing that a diagnosis of AD, even in the moderate to severe stages, does not mean that a person cannot experience a number of indicators of relative well-being, including the ability to care about another person.

Previously in this chapter, I discussed instances in which people with AD acted purposefully to avoid situations they knew to be potentially embarrassing or humiliating to them. Each of those instances revealed the indicators of relative well-being, "self-respect" and the "assertion of desire or will." In Western culture, self-respect is thought to be important. So when a person diagnosed with AD acts in a way to preserve his or her self-respect, it is a positive sign that ought to be appreciated and valued by others for the psychological and brain-related significance (healthy brain systems must be involved in this kind of thinking) that it reflects.

The presence of these indicators of relative well-being is not acknowledged in any way in the standard neuropsychological assessment of cognitive ability that is carried out in the hospital clinic or neuropsychologist's office, and unfortunately, these do not figure into the assessment of the degree of severity of the disease in terms of its stage. This is an arbitrary choice on the part of those making assessments in clinics. Nevertheless, these indicators are extremely valuable abilities in human life regardless of whether or not a person is diagnosed. Indeed, the absence of all of them would render a person quite stunted in his or her interactions with others. Thus, there is all the more reason for care partners to focus their attention carefully so as to observe the presence of these indicators. After all, they mean a great deal more for everyone concerned than does whether or not the person with AD can recall what he or she ate for breakfast earlier in the day, for example. In other words, rather than focusing mainly on what the diagnosed person cannot do at all or on what he or she has trouble doing, care partners need to see what their loved one's strengths still are, not just in general terms but also in very specific terms such as these various indicators of relative well-being. When we can name with precision people's strengths, we come to appreciate those strengths and notice them increasingly more so as to create a more realistic understanding of the person diagnosed. And for the person diagnosed, it means having his or her remaining abilities not only appreciated but also engaged, and this can have very beneficial effects in the life of the person diagnosed and, therefore, in the life of his or her care partner.

In addition to the previously discussed and other indicators of relative well-being, Kitwood (1998) proposed that underlying these indicators are the following "global sentient states":

- The sense of personal worth
- A sense of agency
- Social confidence
- A sense of hope

The logic here is that without these states of being, it would be quite difficult for a person to manifest the indicators of relative well-being. For example, one would not try to help someone if one did not hope that by doing so a positive outcome might occur or if one did not have a sense of confidence or of personal worth. People with dementia of different types can and do express a variety of hopes in life, just as do people not diagnosed, and these are found often to be felt in connection with the well-being of others (Wolverson, Clarke, & Moniz-Cook,

2010). What this means about people with AD was expressed beautifully by Lisa Snyder (2001), who said, "The perseverance of hope can indeed form the bridge that links our common humanity to persons with Alzheimer's" (p. 19).

As mentioned at the outset of this section, the various indicators of relative well-being become apparent in social situations. People with AD and other forms of dementia, and people not diagnosed, live among others and interact with them in a social world. As is the case with all people, those diagnosed with AD or another dementia can be affected for better and for worse by their interactions with others. This is the subject of Chapter 4.

4

PEOPLE WITH ALZHEIMER'S DISEASE AND THE SOCIAL WORLD

Life in the everyday social world can be a very difficult, even foreboding, experience for a person diagnosed with Alzheimer's disease (AD) or another type of dementia, or it can be an experience characterized by acceptance, understanding, and nurturance and can be rewarding despite the losses the person experiences due to brain damage. Whether it is the former or the latter depends tremendously on how others treat the person diagnosed. Interestingly, the same could be said about people who are not diagnosed with AD or another form of dementia. How people deemed healthy treat people with AD or other types of dementia will depend in part on the way they think about aging in general and dementia in particular.

Is there negative stereotyping about aging in general?

Western culture in developed countries seems to harbor negative stereotypic attitudes toward aging (Zhang et al., 2006). For example, one never hears a person say, "I'm having a senior moment" after having said something in a beautifully erudite way that exemplifies love, generosity, wisdom, kindness, gratitude, ethical thought, devotion to the welfare of others, the interdependence of people, or valued principles. Rather, "senior moments" refer to failures of one kind or another—for example, not recalling quickly a particular piece of information such as the name of a famous actor or why one walked into a particular room in the house a moment ago.

This attitude is reflected also in birthday cards. Birthday cards for children and young adults are happy, brightly colored, and replete with expressions of delight and hope, but once people reach the age of 30, 35, and surely 40 years and beyond, the messages are altogether different. Birthday cards for people in midlife announce that they are "over the hill" or "going downhill," and then there are birthday cards for people in their 70s and 80s, in which a question on the cover such as "How's life now that you're 75?" is answered on the inside by "It Depends." The joke here, as it were, is that Depends is the name of an adult diaper. These are the messages that we frequently present to ourselves about aging in a variety of social situations, and they are so powerful that in an informal poll I took in my own classes in recent years, bright undergraduate students in large numbers said that they were afraid of growing old. Although this was admittedly not a scientific effort, it was telling nonetheless.

When people grow up in a climate of negative stereotyping regarding aging and when they themselves become middle-aged and older, they often engage in what social psychologists call "self-stereotyping" (Levy, 1996): They begin to own the negative stereotypes to which they were exposed for years and now apply them to themselves, hence the use of the descriptor "senior moment" for failures of one or another kind. It is as remarkable as it is sad that such a negative expression about aging has become omnipresent in US culture today. An unfortunate result of this situation is known as "stereotype threat," which occurs when older people are made aware that one of their stigmatized attributes, such as their memory, is being tested. Under these conditions, people perform worse than they otherwise would (Barber, Mather, & Gatz, 2015; Steele, 1997), essentially living up to the stereotype, and their poor performance is often interpreted, by those unaware of the effect of stereotype threat, as being due to their age rather than to the social circumstances in which they were tested. So we have a situation in which aging is thought of negatively in general. Added to this are the remarkably negative stereotypes about dementia in general and AD in particular.

Is there negative stereotyping about Alzheimer's disease and dementia even among professionals?

Surprisingly, yes. For example, in referring to people with AD in a book titled *Enhancing the Quality of Life in Advanced Dementia*, a very well-meaning professional wrote, "Even if the patient is given the most logical, eloquent argument why he or she should not go outside [in a rainstorm], there is nothing in his or her brain that can appreciate the reasoning" (Raia, 1999, p. 31). There is no substantive scientific evidence to support this statement. Another example from the same book is the following: "In a long-term study . . . nurses reported that patients receiving validation therapy were less physically and verbally aggressive, less depressed, but more non-physically aggressive in terms of increased wandering, pacing, and repetitive movement" (Benjamin, 1999, p. 124). What is it about a person walking that makes it "wandering"? Who wanders? Who takes a walk? If one has a diagnosis of dementia, does the act of walking suddenly become wandering, even "aimless" wandering, and if so, why? Are nursing home residents unable to take a walk? Must they wander? What is it about walking, pacing, or making repetitive movements that makes those actions "aggressive" in any way? Imagine people in a hospital waiting area pacing back and forth while awaiting news of a loved one's operation and being asked why they are being so "non-physically aggressive." They would be completely within reason if they responded with stunned, quizzical, silence at the obvious absurdity of the question. If describing pacing as "non-physically aggressive" is absurd in the case of people in a hospital waiting room, why is it not absurd in the case of a nursing home resident diagnosed with advanced dementia? The following is a final example (Benjamin, 1999):

> Patients in the second stage are increasingly disoriented as to time, place, and person. The patients who are time-confused are no longer anxious, but rather are unfocused . . . are difficult to motivate and will not conform to the expectations of family and staff. (pp. 113–114)

No one can logically or scientifically assert that another person is not anxious if the person's discourse—what he or she says and does—reflects anxiety. The tests of orientation typically employed demand recall of information, and as mentioned previously, recall is the method of retrieval from memory that is most negatively affected by dementia. People diagnosed are rarely, if ever, given the opportunity to retrieve information about orientation in other ways. Furthermore, if such people are living in a nursing home and rarely, if ever, leave, why would one assume that it would be important for them to keep in mind what day of the week it is or what month it is or what year it is? Finally, what exactly are the "expectations" of staff to which the person does not "conform"? The point here is that even among professionals, horrifically negative stereotypes exist regarding persons with dementia, and one must wonder how such attitudes and beliefs affect how these professionals treat persons diagnosed and, hence, the way the persons diagnosed react.

With this as background, it was unsurprising that Dr. M, a brilliant social scientist, was reluctant to tell her adult children and close friends about her diagnosis for quite some time. She reflected on this in a speech she gave to social workers a year after her diagnosis:

> Why this reluctance to name my malady? Can it be that the term, "Alzheimer's" has a connotation similar to the

"Scarlett Letter" or the "Black Plague"? Is it even more embarrassing than a sexual disease? At any rate, the order in which I came to "tell all" to friends, to say that I had AD had a lot to do with my feeling of "being safe" with the friend.

Dr. M's experience is similar in a way to that of Jean, diagnosed with AD, who said the following about her ability to speak fluently with other people (Snyder, 2009):

> There is embarrassment when I want to say, "ocean" and I can't think of the word. It depends on how comfortable I am with the person I'm talking with. … There is the issue of safety. If I'm in a group of women with whom I am comfortable, I'm not as likely to have a problem. But if it's somebody that I don't know, then I feel like I'm practically scaring them. (p. 62)

Finally, Betty, also diagnosed with AD, noted,

> People may deny that they have Alzheimer's disease because they don't have the opportunity to talk with other people who are sympathetic and understanding and who will help them along in the whole process. Anyone who has this diagnosis needs to have others with whom to talk. (p. 120)

What prevents people with Alzheimer's disease or another dementia from feeling safe in social situations?

Tom Kitwood (1998) asserted that how people think about and act toward those diagnosed can be "malignant," or dangerous. This is the case because these forms of thought and action can depersonalize people diagnosed and assault their feelings of self-worth, leading them to feel unworthy and burdensome and hurt. Kitwood termed these actions "malignant social psychology," and he provided examples of a host of ways in which those deemed healthy act to the detriment of those diagnosed. It is especially important to note that Kitwood was quite clear that these and other forms of malignant social psychology are enacted quite innocently, for no one acts in these ways toward another person with malicious intent. Due to their very limited understanding about people with dementia, healthy care partners assume incorrectly that what they are doing is not harmful to the person diagnosed. The following is not to be thought of as a complete list, but it surely illuminates many actions to be avoided by professional and informal care partners if they want to help the person diagnosed to feel safe:

1. *Treachery*: Using deception to distract or manipulate a person or force them into compliance. For example, Mrs. W, a nursing home resident diagnosed with AD, does not want to get dressed in the morning, so an aide lies to her, telling her that she needs to get dressed because her son is coming to take her home later in the morning. Mrs. W then gets dressed, but she also packs a suitcase with some clothes and goes to the lobby and sits there waiting for her son to arrive. As Mrs. W sits in the lobby waiting, another aide tells her that she has to come to a particular room for an activity. Mrs. W tells the aide that her son is coming to take her home and that she wants to wait for him in the lobby rather than go elsewhere. The aide knows that this is not the case and, unaware of the lie Mrs. W was told earlier by another aide, assumes that Mrs. W is being delusional, harboring a false belief, said to be a psychiatric symptom of AD.

2. *Disempowerment*: Not allowing a person to use the abilities he or she still has; not helping the person to complete actions already initiated. An aide feeds a nursing home resident because it would take more time if the resident fed herself. The resident thereby gradually stops feeding

herself when she has the opportunity to do so. In another example, Mr. K does not let his wife set the dinner table even though she is willing and able to do so, and so she sits and does nothing. She is then said to be apathetic, doing none of the things around the house that she did years ago.

3. *Infantilization*: Treating a person very patronizingly as an insensitive parent might treat a young child. Examples include using "elderspeak" and speaking to a person as if he or she were a child in a "sing-song" way.

4. *Intimidation*: Inducing fear in a person through the use of threats or physical power. Gen. U, a nursing home resident, did not want to take a shower at 7 a.m. when an aide told him that it was time to do so. Eventually, after repeatedly telling Gen. U it is time to take a shower and Gen. U refusing to get out of bed, the aide tries to pull Mr. U out of his bed, thereby applying force. Gen. U resists physically, hitting the aide, and is then described as being combative and uncooperative. Interestingly, Gen U, as a nursing home resident, has lost the right to take a shower at a time of his choosing.

5. *Labeling*: Using the diagnosis as the main basis for interacting with a person and for explaining his or her actions. Mrs. D was angry with her husband because he unwittingly humiliated her in front of day center staff members by tucking her turtleneck top into her slacks (although she looked fine). Later that evening, Mr. D became aware of his wife's anger, as she did not speak to him or look at him, and he referred subsequently to her anger as "irrational hostility," which indicated to him that, as he said, "the Alzheimer's is getting worse." This is a fine example also of how the diagnosis changes a great deal about our understanding of interpersonal interactions. In the normal, everyday world, if Person A acts angrily toward Person B and Person B does not know why, Person B will be confused but will not accuse Person A of being "irrationally hostile." Person B may ask, "Why are you angry

with me?" But as soon as Person A has a diagnosis of AD or some other form of dementia, Person B's lack of understanding of why Person A is angry becomes transformed into Person A being "irrationally angry" or "irrationally hostile." In other words, Person B is essentially saying the following about the person diagnosed: "Because I do not understand why he or she is angry with me, he or she must be irrational." Why do the "rules of engagement" or "rules of understanding" change so dramatically when a person has a diagnosis of AD? When I pointed out to Mr. D that he inadvertently humiliated his wife publicly, he was clearly terribly sorry, saying, "Doc, you have to believe me. I'd never do anything to hurt her; I love her." I believed him completely. I had no doubt at all about the deep love he felt for his wife and that he meant no harm whatsoever. This is a clear example of how malignant social psychology is not malicious or intentional.

6. *Stigmatization*: The exclusion of the person diagnosed so that he or she becomes an outcast. Mrs. K had a number of siblings, and they and their spouses lived close by. For years, they gathered on Friday evenings for dinner at one or another's home. After Mrs. K was diagnosed, she and her husband were no longer invited, and when they invited others to their home, the others always had other plans. Interestingly, Mrs. K was put on an antidepressant medication even though the reason for her sadness was clear and did not go away. The reason for her sadness involved the way her relatives treated her, and that continued even though she was medicated. Just the same, her sadness was interpreted as a symptom of AD rather than a symptom of being treated so badly by her relatives who were, as are so many people, deeply afraid of being with people diagnosed with AD. This attitude is reflected in Bea's comment, "We've never tried to hide the fact that I have Alzheimer's. But everyone acts like they don't want to get near because they might catch it" (Snyder, 2009, p. 24).

7. *Outpacing*: Occurs when others go about doing things at a speed that is too rapid for the diagnosed person. Thus, the person is left out of conversations because he or she cannot think and speak quickly enough to match the rate of otherwise healthy others.

8. *Invalidation*: The denial of, overlooking, or ignoring the subjectivity of the person with dementia. For example, if the person with dementia is anxious about something, the anxiety is viewed as symptomatic of dementia rather than being a reaction to a situation that exists in the social world. Thus, no attempt is made to provide the person with sensitive support, and no attempt is made to do something about the situation that inspired the feeling because the anxiety is viewed as a symptom of disease rather than a reaction to something real in the person's experience. In connection with an experience different from anxiety but still an example of invalidation, Mr. D claimed that "the maids overindulge my wife" (diagnosed with AD) because they give her an afghan when she says she is cold in the house. This is "overindulging" because Mr. D says that it is not cold in the house, given that he does not feel cold. Therefore, in his view, his wife says she feels cold because of AD and is therefore incorrect about her own experience of feeling cold.

9. *Banishment*: Others avoid the person diagnosed, who is viewed as "confused" and worthy of removal from the social world of others. Betty, the retired social worker, noted, "Now Alzheimer's disease has a lot of attention, and the symptoms that are described scare people—that we'll walk blindly into a car because we're lost and wandering. It isn't necessarily true, but people get an idea" (Snyder, 2009, p. 120). Indeed, it is quite common for people to withdraw their friendship from those diagnosed, and this adds to the diagnosed person's feelings of depression and abandonment (Harris, 2004; Harris & Keady, 2004; Snyder, 2009; Sterin, 2002). In addition to the psychological and emotional effects, the social isolation

(lack of friendship) experienced by people diagnosed can include poor quality of life in terms of physical health (Hawthorne, 2006).

10. *Objectification*: The person diagnosed is not treated as someone worthy of respect or simple common courtesy; he or she is talked about in uncomplimentary ways and is thought of as "an AD patient" or a "dysfunctional or burdensome dementia patient" rather than as a person.

11. *Ignoring*: Healthy others carry on a conversation, even about the person diagnosed, in the presence of that person as if he or she were not there. This utterly disrespectful behavior would never be inflicted on a person deemed healthy.

12. *Imposition*: Forcing a diagnosed person to do something without giving the person a choice. Mrs. L, who is a nursing home resident, is seated in a wheelchair and is having a conversation with someone. A staff member arrives and tells Mrs. L that it is time for lunch and abruptly wheels her away from her partner in conversation without allowing her to finish what she was saying or to choose to finish her conversation before going to lunch. She continues talking louder and louder as she is wheeled away from her interlocutor.

13. *Withholding*: The refusal to provide attention when it is requested to meet a real need.

14. *Accusation*: Blaming the person with dementia for doing something or failing to do something as a result of his or her inability or due to the person having misunderstood the situation. A family care partner accuses the person with AD of deliberately not recalling what he or she was told 5 minutes ago or deliberately not putting something where it truly belongs simply to annoy or hurt the care partner.

15. *Mockery*: Making jokes at the expense of the person diagnosed.

16. *Disparagement*: Telling the person diagnosed that he or she is burdensome or incompetent. Referring to the person as "demented" falls into this category because the

definition of demented is to be without a mind, insane, and the like. A person diagnosed with dementia is neither of these.

17. *Disruption*: Interrupting the person abruptly in the midst of doing something such as speaking, thereby breaking up the person's "frame of reference" in Kitwood's (1998) words.

It should be clear that treating people with AD or another type of dementia in these ways constitutes an assault on their feelings of self-worth and depersonalizes them. It is akin to pouring salt on an open wound, exacerbating the effects of the brain damage caused by the disease, and prevents the person from feeling "safe" in social situations. Under these conditions, it is not surprising that many people diagnosed with dementia of any type react by withdrawing from social situations further and experiencing deep, damaging isolation. This reaction would not be a symptom of dementia in general or of AD in particular but, rather, a reaction to being treated in a socially dysfunctional way. Indeed, avoiding such social situations would be a rather logical adaptation to feeling unsafe, maligned, and hurt. If a person with dementia reacted this way, it would be a sign of self-respect as well as an assertion of will—two of Kitwood's (1998) indicators of relative well-being that were discussed in Chapter 3. Would any of us wish to be in a situation that was demeaning or hurtful, in which we were not treated with the common courtesy we experienced for decades of adult life? It would be rather self-destructive not to avoid such treatment.

How can one help the person diagnosed to feel safe?

One obvious answer is not to act in ways that could be characterized as malignant social psychology, but although that is very important, it is only the first step. Other steps that are helpful are discussed next.

1. *Taking the intentional stance (Dennett, 1988) toward the person diagnosed*: This means that we view what the person does or says as an attempt to communicate something even if that something is unclear to us. That is, we assume that the person with dementia has thoughts, feelings, attitudes, and beliefs that he or she wants to share despite his or her word-finding or other language-related problems. The fact that what the person means may not be clear to the listener does not mean that the person is not trying to say something meaningful or important. If I do not understand what the person with dementia says, he or she is not "confused." Rather, I am! My goal, therefore, is to seek to understand what the person is trying to say or to give the person the opportunity to act before assuming that his or her actions are dysfunctional.

For example, at an adult day center, Mr. R, who was diagnosed with AD, opened the wardrobe in which participants' coats were hung during the day and, beginning at one end and moving systematically toward the other, one at a time, took things out of the pockets of each coat, looked at them, and then put them back. He did this repeatedly until he came to a particular coat, looked at the contents, put them back, and took that coat off the hanger and put it on. It was his coat. It would have been easy for a staff member to interpret this seemingly inappropriate action as a completely dysfunctional, purposeless result of AD. Instead, she allowed him to continue and saw the result. Mr. R could not recognize his coat from among the rest, but he could recognize his "stuff" in the pockets, so this was an adaptation and a successful one at that. He was clearly intending to find his coat and was using the only means at his disposal to do so. His action was not, in itself, pathological or meaningless. Rather, it was a clear, goal-directed action even if it was not the usual way to identify one's coat; we generally do not examine others' property without permission.

An example of taking the intentional stance when a person with dementia is speaking was presented in Chapter 3: Mr. R was speaking to me with great urgency and agitation, and I did not understand what he was trying to say even though he was speaking words that, individually, were coherent. I assumed that he was trying to tell me something meaningful. I did not assume that he was confused simply because I did not understand what he was saying, any more than I would assume someone speaking a language I did not understand to be confused. I felt great compassion for him because he was obviously deeply upset and was trying desperately to communicate something he felt to be important. So I focused on the obvious fact that he was very upset and asked him, "Do you feel like crying?" And, with eyes wide open, he replied with the first coherent sentence I heard, "You're damn right I do!" In engaging Mr. R this way, I communicated to him that I was listening to him—hearing more than just the words he was speaking, but also the emotional tone he was exhibiting and trying to work with him in what might be called a "joint venture" to figure out what he was trying to communicate. This, in turn, provided him with the confidence that I was listening actively to and caring about what he was saying, and that allowed him to feel safe with me.

2. *Actively listening in conversation*: The next step after taking the intentional stance is to engage in active listening, which can occur during any conversation between people who share an interest in a topic and who care about communicating clearly with one another. When we truly care about our partner in conversation, we give him or her our focused attention, and if we are not sure we understand what he or she is saying, we say so. Or, for example, if the person is talking about a painful situation, we might commiserate and say, "Gosh that had to have been so difficult for you to go through, especially on that day." In other words, we do not say, "Uh-huh" in the flat-toned, vacant way, usually uttered at the wrong time, that we hear when someone with whom we are speaking on the phone is paying attention to what is on his or her computer screen instead of what we are saying. That is passive, unfocused, uninterested listening.

Another response that fails to qualify as active listening often occurs in a situation such as the one with Mr. R, in which the listener has no idea what the speaker means and, instead of exploring what is behind the emotional urgency and distress, responds by saying, "Okay, okay, calm down" or something along those lines. By saying "Okay," the speaker is communicating that he or she understands what the person diagnosed is saying, when the opposite is true. So active listening involves responding honestly and earnestly to what one's partner in conversation is saying or is trying to say. When we do not understand what a person with AD is saying, we should not say "okay" or "uh-huh." We should say, "I'm having trouble understanding what you're saying" because that is the truth. Better yet is saying with great sincerity, "I'm having trouble understanding what you're saying, and I need your help."

Another approach is observed in the case of Mrs. F, who had great linguistic difficulties but who was a very expressive person who participated in many plays and taught acting and other performing arts. One way to work with her when having difficulty understanding what she was saying was to say "Show me," and she would then act out what she was trying to convey previously through words alone (Sabat & Cagigas, 1997).

Conversations are types of contracts between people, each of whom takes responsibility for what happens in the communicative act and is willing to cooperate with the other to achieve clear communication. When one person has linguistic difficulties, the other person retains responsibility to elucidate what the speaker is trying to say and may have to expend considerable effort. One might say that active listening is akin to playing detective, trying to find the answer to the question, What is this person trying to tell me? Another way to find the answer is to use what linguists call indirect repair (De Bleser & Weisman, 1986).

3. *Using indirect repair in conversation*: Let me explain this first by comparing it with direct repair. Direct repair occurs often when a teacher corrects a student's grammatical error or mispronunciation of a word. In this case, the teacher repairs the student's speech. Indirect repair is repairing the listener's understanding of what the speaker says when the

listener does not clearly understand the speaker's statement. The listener can use indirect repair in a few different ways. One is to check with the speaker to determine if the listener has understood what the speaker has said by stating, for example, "I'm not sure that I understand what you're saying, so let me see if I do. You are saying that . . .," at which point the listener says what he or she thinks the speaker meant originally. The speaker can then say "yes" or "no" or "close." Now the listener can try again, questioning what the speaker intended. The following example demonstrates my use of indirect repair with Dr. M. She was talking about her experience of being tested by a speech therapist and her decision not to pursue speech therapy. The numbers in parentheses indicate my use of indirect repair (Sabat, 1991, p. 291):

DR. M: I had three days, no, times and on the third day I told her (the speech therapist) that I would have to give up the program. It was, and she wanted very much to know why, and I said uh, that uh, I have too many things on my head and they aren't, don't fit together or something like that. At any rate, that's not something that's helping me uh, if, and then she—before we're going away, you will tell me what you feel about this. (Shows me the results of the tests.)

SRS: Well, I'm familiar with some of the tests that they gave you.

DR. M: And uh, this was at the time, it was about three weeks ago and um, I was doing other things and it didn't, it didn't give me a feeling that there's something that I should have another thing.

SRS: It didn't give you the feeling that going back and doing some kind of speech therapy would be helpful to you? (1)

DR. M: No, I didn't think about that and uh, I, d, it wasn't, it wasn't important and I, you know, at this time too, I found that I really don't like to be uh, talking about what, what's my trouble. It's gotten, I know what my trouble is. And I think that what I would like it uh, only if there's something that is, uh, a time, a uh, a time and with a person who there is a real (gestures with hands, holding them vertically in front of her, parallel to one another about 5 inches apart and moving the right hand toward the left hand and then the left hand toward the right hand back and forth repeatedly)

SRS: Back and forth—a relationship. (2)

DR. M: Um hum. You know you could go out, out of this area, and you could get so many people who would want to, to for one reason or another, to do uh, something uh, with me, and I don't want that. I don't want my life to be uh, not uh, I don't want to be part of what does this person can do, what that person do.

SRS: Let me back up for a second because I think I'm missing your point. You don't want your life to be (3)

DR. M: Going always to see people to see what's wrong with me.

SRS: Ah!

DR. M: And how to, and how and how it could sometimes uh, what can we do about it? But otherwise, I've, I've, I've had it.

SRS: Ya ... let me see if I understand. At least one of the things that you're saying is that it's, it's not something you, you don't want to put yourself in situations where you're constantly being shown what you can't do. (4)

DR. M: That's one. That a real thing.

In this part of a longer conversation, I worked diligently with Dr. M to try to repair my understanding of what she was trying to tell me, and she and I worked together to elucidate why she did not want to continue with speech therapy. She and I had a coherent conversation even though she had serious word-finding problems. We learn that she quite logically does not want to put herself in a position to see what is wrong with her all the time. This is an example of self-respect and an assertion of will, both of which are among Kitwood's (1998) indicators of relative well-being. In this conversation, we see also that she would prefer to have a social relationship with another person that is enlivening rather than spending time interacting with a professional person in a patient–professional type of relationship. We can thus appreciate how indirect repair can be used to help understand the subjective experience of the person with AD.

Dr. M's husband, a brilliant person as well, was frustrated because he did not understand why his wife did not want to continue seeing the speech therapist. In order to reach that level of understanding, it was imperative to use indirect repair to learn what going to the speech therapist meant to Dr. M and, therefore, why she found it so aversive. In this sense, she acted quite logically: No one enjoys being shown repeatedly what he or she cannot do. This is especially true if the things one cannot do are personally very important. Furthermore, being a very social person, Dr. M wanted to have social relationships with people and that was becoming increasingly difficult due to her diagnosis. Under these circumstances, she did not want virtually all of her social relationships to be focused on testing and assessment and being shown repeatedly the degree to which she had lost her previous level of linguistic ability. Note that using indirect repair requires one to be listening actively.

Why do active listening and taking the intentional stance help the person with dementia feel safe?

When we take the intentional stance, listen actively, and employ indirect repair, we convey to people with AD or another type of dementia that we are deeply interested in and committed to communicating with them so as to learn what they want to say. This is truly a form of honoring the person diagnosed as a human being worthy of another person's time and effort for the sole purpose of being with and learning from him or her. These are overt expressions of great caring and concern, and people diagnosed are very sensitive to and appreciative of the positive meaning implicit in this form of interaction, as would be anyone deemed healthy. Mispronunciations and errors in syntax are not highlighted. Rather than diminishing their sense of self-worth as do forms of malignant social psychology, these forms of interaction enhance the feelings of self-worth of people with AD, giving them the sense that "this person cares about listening to me and understanding me." It is important to remember that people with AD or other dementias are extremely vulnerable, given their sense of personal losses and the resulting sadness, anger, frustration, grief, and loneliness that they often experience.

These feelings are reflected in an interaction I had with Dr. B. At one point in our association, which lasted 9 months of meeting twice a week for 2 hours at a time, Dr. B asked, "What keeps you going about me?" For a person to ask such a question reveals the need for reassurance that there is something about the person worthy of the interest that I expressed and the time I spent with him or her and of the work that we did together. For Dr. B to have asked that question also reveals his own feeling of being safe—safe enough to ask and to hear the answer. His feeling of vulnerability is quite clear in the following conversational extract:

DR. B: So—are you going to throw me out of the shed?
SRS: Not me. Not for a minute. Are you kidding? (I took his question to mean, "Are you going to stop working with me?" or "Are you going to end my work on The Project?")
DR. B: What keeps you going about me?
SRS: What keeps me going about you? Now there's a question! You mean why do I keep coming and talking with you and doing this? (Note the use of indirect repair here.)
DR. B: Um hum.
SRS: I think that you have a lot to teach about the effects of Alzheimer's, especially in terms of the things you can still do. The person who has the disease is not, in my opinion, well understood. I want to change that with your help. It's a matter of human dignity.

DR. B: Well, I got a lot of dignity.

SRS: You certainly do. I want also to show that the person with Alzheimer's can learn new things, can remember new things, over a long period of time.

DR. B: Um hum. What I want I think I've got. I've got that you have stayed with me. I have a lot of feeling for my family and, uh, so I'm hoping you can stay with me.

The need to be accepted and to enjoy honest, open communication and also to be treated as an equal is common to most human beings and it is, as it turns out, a need felt by people with AD and other types of dementia as well.

This need was evident also in a study on the effectiveness and value of support groups for people with mild to moderate AD (Snyder, Jenkins, & Joosten, 2007). Almost one-fourth of the 70 participants in the survey indicated that they attended group meetings primarily for the companionship and socialization offered, more than one-fifth said they came to learn and to help them cope with the diagnosis or memory problems, and others came to be with people who had the same problems related to AD. One member tellingly reported, "To be with a group that feels the same as I do and has the same problems. I don't feel strange about revealing what is going on with me" (p. 17), thereby affirming the importance of feeling accepted. Among the things they liked best about the group were that the group felt like a family and that there was a sense of friendship and companionship among the members—a sense that provided a feeling of being safe. One person commented about the group, "The positive attitude. It's uplifting. The reason for being here is not funny, but everyone is laughing" (p. 17). Twenty percent of the participants said that the verbal sharing or learning they experienced was the part of the group they liked best. One person said, "When we can share things and then that way we might be able to help each other" (p. 17). Only in a setting in which people feel safe can they enjoy such feelings and the ability to speak openly and honestly about what matters most to them. People in such groups listen actively to one another and work cooperatively to clarify what they mean with the words they speak if they are not being clearly understood by others in the group. In a sense, the support group mirrors what happens among any group of people who gather for a common purpose. None of the people experiences anything remotely resembling malignant social psychology in these settings, and so they feel safe and exult in the personal connections they develop as a result. No one stands in harsh judgment if a group member fails to recall something or mispronounces a word, so there is a certain calm shared among the group members, which is another important aspect of a safe environment.

4. *Providing a non-anxious presence*: People with AD or other types of dementia can often find themselves in situations that are upsetting, aggravating, or even scary. For example, Bea (Snyder, 2009) spoke about a number of things that are troublesome to her:

> And money! Money is getting to be terrible. Just don't want to handle money anymore because I can't identify it. (p. 23)
>
> I don't like to make mistakes. I get aggravated with myself, and I can cry a lot easier than I can laugh. I would rather live with better feelings than I have at times. I'd like to be perfect. But I never have been and never will be. This disease makes you feel so helpless. I've lost my feeling of self-satisfaction that I was capable of doing things, and I resent it a little bit. But I'll live through it. (p. 27)
>
> I can feed myself to a point. But I have a hard time identifying the food. I can see it, but I can't tell what it is. So it's a hassle. (p. 30)

When people live much of each day with feelings such as these, the last thing they need is to be in the presence of someone who is a fountain of anxiety in reaction to what it is that the person with AD is doing or failing to do. As is true for most people who are not diagnosed, being in the presence of others who are calm can have a calming effect on people with dementia, allowing them to do things better than they might otherwise be able. So providing a non-anxious presence is something that can help the person with dementia feel safe, for being diagnosed with AD or another type of dementia does not mean that the person is insensitive to the emotional tone exhibited by what others say and do.

There are times, however, when the circumstances facing the person diagnosed can be even more troubling. This kind of situation and the virtue of a non-anxious presence are exemplified well in a situation in which three students in my advanced seminar in clinical neuropsychology—Anila D'Mello, Lina Jamis, and Jessie Schwab—found themselves when riding on the Washington, DC, subway. They were on their way to the adult day center for their final 3-hour visit of the semester. What happened is beautifully captured in Anila's journal entry for the course that day. Anila was well versed in aspects of biology and chemistry in addition to psychology, Lina was a senior pre-medical student who did volunteer emergency medicine work, and Jessie was a psychology major who would go on to graduate school. In this entry, we find the students, having learned about the effects of brain injury in the course and from the people with whom they interacted at the adult day center, encountering a woman with dementia on the subway and going about helping her, all the while providing a non-anxious presence:

We never made it to the Center today; however, the experience we had was relevant, touching, and unforgettable. As our train pulled up to a stop only a few stops from our final destination, Jessie, Lina, and I watched attentively as an elderly lady with a walker approached a sleeping passenger and shook her forcefully to wake her up.

"I don't know where I am," the elderly lady announced to no one in particular, looking around in confusion. Her confusion seemed more than an inquiry about which stop the train was approaching and the three of us jumped up to talk to her. "I don't know where I am. I don't know where I'm going," the lady repeated to us. Lina instantly had an idea. "Would you like to look at the map? Maybe some of these names will jog your memory." The lady seemed tired, inattentive, and agitated at her inability to recognize her surroundings. Lina tried again, noticing the suitcase situated on her walker, " 'It looks like you're traveling?" We coaxed her to sit down and discussed a few strategies with her that might help her remember where she was meant to go. The originally sleeping woman, unmoving and seemingly unconcerned, tsked ("tsk, tsk") a few times and shook her head, "That's dementia. She has dementia. First it's the short term memory then it's the long term memory." I was instantly angered. Unhelpful and in fact harmful, this woman was only further distressing our elderly lady. I asked the elderly lady for her name, "Anne" she replied. We assured her that we wouldn't leave her, that we would stay with her as long as she needed us. Meanwhile, Anne repeatedly smacked her hand against her head, "There is something wrong," she said, "This is not right." She had a slight German accent and her protestations seemed to imply that these "memory-lapses" were not usual for her. In addition, this negative reaction towards her inability to recall certain details reassured me that Anne *did have* all the information we needed in order to get her to the right place—it was only a matter of accessing it. She rifled through her purse, checking and re-checking pockets and scraps of paper before suddenly looking up with a start, "A train. I'm supposed to be on a train." With this information in working memory, Anne dove into her purse and extracted a yellow notepad with written information. It was as if understanding *what* her purpose was also enabled her to *find* what it was she needed. We examined the notepad:

South Carelina (sic.)

9:55 AM

Florence

Apparently, Anne was supposed to have been on a train heading to South Carolina, one that she had missed (it was now 10:00 AM). "Union Station?" We exclaimed, "Is that where you are supposed to be?" Anne nodded and like that, we had a destination. Some arguments ensued with the suddenly interested sleeping lady in the corner. "Keep her on the train till the end of the line and then it'll turn around to Union. She's confused. She has dementia." . . . The woman seemed irritated with my behavior and dismissal of her comments of Anne's mental states, "You don't even *know* how to deal with people with dementia" she said to me. I snapped. "Actually, we're all certified to deal with people with dementia," I retorted (shouldn't have lied), and focused on Anne. As she rifled through her purse, I noticed a few important things. One was a small black case, similar to the one I have often seen in the possession of diabetics. The second was a slender telephone book. I jumped up, "Can I see that telephone book, Anne?" She willingly gave it to us. While slowing the process, having her permission before seeing and touching her things seemed like the right thing to do to avoid any further distress or confusion on her part. I flipped through the book while Lina asked her yes or no questions concerning her family and purpose in going to South Carolina. This information was sufficient in enabling us to find a few names and numbers of relatives to call. I noted one in particular with an address in Alexandria, VA. "Who is James, Anne? Can we call him?" I asked. Her eyes got wide and she pulled the book away from me and put it back into her

purse. Luckily, Lina had jotted down the telephone number of Anne's South Carolina son. The train progressed
towards Union Station as we attempted multiple times to
call her son. "He won't answer. He can't," she said time
and time again, not able to explain exactly why this was
the case. Her hands shaking, she removed the diabetes
case from her purse attempting to open it to measure
her blood sugar. Unfortunately, her hands were shaking uncontrollably and she was unable to draw blood
with which to get a reading on her monitor. This was the
only point throughout the day that I decided to act forcefully rather than waiting for permission. After multiple
failed attempts, I removed the blood-drawing tool from
her hand while Lina held her hand steady and prepared
the monitor. I pricked her finger, feeling relieved as the
blood trickled into the monitor which flashed a "53" on
the screen. That was low. Once again, I slightly over-
stepped boundaries as I asked Anne if she had any food
with my hand already searching the grocery bag on her
walker. She consented and I found orange juice, sugar
packets, and various other snacks that I knew (from previous dealings with diabetics) would efficiently raise her
blood sugar. After downing the drinks and snacks, she
seemed to calm down. Her shaking stopped, her color
improved and she was able to answer our questions
robustly. She explained that James of Alexandria was her
ex-husband and that her son was enlisted in the military.
I thanked the preparation I had received in this course
that I had not hastily made a call to James and listened
to her instead.

Soon we arrived at Union Station. The yellow "M"
on the sugar packets I had originally found in a panic
prompted me to ask her if she would like McDonald's.
She nodded, "That's my thing." Things were coming
together. Our relative calm had paid off and Anne was
relaxed and able to help us help her. We had reached her

daughter-in-law who gave us further direction in terms of re-booking a train ticket, etc. From then on, the day went smoothly. She was booked for a 7 PM train and all she had to do was wait.

Today was exhausting. I was anxious and at times hasty. Nonetheless, I was blessed to have had capable friends who kept me calm (Lina sent me a text saying, "Non anxious presence" at one point). I was surprised at the amount of *knowledge* we had from this course, from previous encounters with friends, from other experiences that enabled us to effectively deal with problems that arose, emotional and medical alike. Mostly, I was impressed with Anne. I was reminded that we all hold the knowledge, the ability to help ourselves within us. It takes some prying, some willingness of others to help . . . but in the end it was Anne who told us everything we needed to know. It was Anne who helped us. I can't imagine a more perfect book-end to this course . . . or, for that matter, this semester. On a personal note, Anne reminded me that everything will be okay (as a graduating senior it's often hard to remember that things will turn out the way they turn out) . . . even in the most confusing times. She reminded me to put my faith in *people* and *humanity* in the most trying moments.

By remaining calm and providing a non-anxious presence, the students were able to help Anne to feel safe and remain calm. That the students took the intentional stance with Anne and essentially played detective in piecing together the story of where Anne was supposed to go was key in this situation. As it turned out, Anne's daughter-in-law phoned the students later in the day to tell them that Anne had arrived safely and to thank them profusely for being so wonderfully kind and helpful. When people feel alone, anxious, and vulnerable, the calm, reassuring presence of others can be of great value in helping them to feel safe. Feeling safe, in turn, allows them to think more clearly than they would if they were in the grip of great anxiety. Family can provide that calm reassurance, but good friends are able to do this very well in rather different ways.

It is already clear that people with AD and other dementias are frequently isolated socially. It is also clear that healthy others can feel very uncomfortable being with those who are diagnosed, even if the person diagnosed is a friend; it is very difficult witnessing the changes that have occurred in some of their friend's attributes, characteristics. Thus, one question that has frequently been asked by people who know someone who has been diagnosed is discussed next.

How can I be a friend to someone with Alzheimer's disease?

One way to begin answering this very important question is to encourage people to employ the various techniques that help the person diagnosed to feel safe and to eliminate all traces of malignant social psychology from our interactions. To answer this question further, though, it seems logical to ask the question, "How can one be a friend to anyone?" After all, persons diagnosed were not always diagnosed with dementia, and they had friends and were friends to others for decades. So let us explore some of what being a friend means, keeping in mind that there is not any single universally accepted definition of friendship.

A provisional, albeit hardly complete, list is as follows:

- Friends provide comfort, understanding, and other help in difficult times.
- They enjoy moments together—walking, listening to music, discussing mutual interests, discussing matters of concern to each, telling stories, making jokes, laughing, watching films, and reveling in each other's joys.
- They support a friend's valued qualities, encourage their expression, and appreciate the person for who he or she is and has been.
- They provide a non-anxious presence when the person needs to express concerns, anxieties, and the like.

Sometimes, they do so by just listening carefully and commiserating while allowing the person to do most of the talking—to "ventilate" as Dr. B said.

- Friends make eye contact when speaking with one another in person.
- Friends understand, or seek to understand, the other's point of view and feelings, and they accept the other's point of view as being quite real.
- Friends celebrate together, show and feel loyalty to one another, trust each other, laugh together, cry together, and break bread together.
- They realize that they cannot always make things all better for the other but try to help the other weather difficulties.
- They apologize sincerely when they have hurt the other person.

In addition to these aspects of friendship, there are specific ways in which one can be a friend to someone with AD or another type of dementia:

- Understand and acknowledge the person's strengths while understanding his or her limitations and finding ways to work around them.
- Remember the capabilities model discussed in Chapter 1.
- Recognize that the person's fundamental values have not changed and help the person maintain those values.
- Treat the person as a whole individual who is not defined entirely by a diagnosis; that is, the person is more than an "dementia patient" and should not be referred to that way.
- Reject mass media-perpetuated distortions and negative stereotypes and stigma associated with dementia in general and AD in particular.
- A person with dementia does not have "memory loss" and can make new memories. If the person does not recall having asked a question a few moments earlier, there is no need to call attention to that fact. Just answer the question as if it were the first time it was asked. This

is a perfect time to provide a non-anxious presence. You can also use the "take a guess" approach after having answered a repeatedly asked question.

- Make good moments, or at least try to do so. The person with dementia can still make new memories because implicit memory systems in the brain can be healthy even if explicit systems, especially those involving conscious recall of recent events, are dysfunctional. Creating good moments will be helpful for the person diagnosed as well as for those otherwise healthy. Life, after all, consists of many, many moments.
- Understand that the person diagnosed needs acceptance. What does the diagnosis mean to the person? Find out, if possible.
- Remind the person with AD that you are still there and will be—that you want to be a friend and make it a point to show that that is true.

Are friendships important to people with Alzheimer's disease or another dementia?

Yes. Harris (2012) examined friendships in the lives of eight people diagnosed with early stage dementia, seven with the Alzheimer's type. It was clear that friendships were important to all eight. One woman noted, "My life depends upon my friends. I really like having people around and being by yourself is not good." Another noted, "If I am going out with a friend or one calls me up, I get undepressed." Clearly, there are good ways to counteract depression that do not involve drugs. Harris also inquired into the factors that are important in a relationship with friends. Among the responses she received from people diagnosed were "The key is being comfortable (with friends). They know what I need. They treat me just like normal"; "My friends don't put me down. A lot of other people think I'm crazy"; and "I make a lot of mistakes and my friends tell me and that is fine. But my, but my friends don't tell me what to do" (p. 309).

One difference between being a patient and being a person is that patients are recipients of care, whereas persons can be givers of care as well as recipients. Many people who are not diagnosed treasure having the opportunity to be of help to others, and many people diagnosed with AD or other types of dementia do so as well. For example, in Harris's (2012) study, one woman commented quite clearly,

> I am a member of a bereavement group and I have been going for a few years. I have made a friend there. After the meetings, we would sit and talk. I like helping people and I am a good listener. It's developed into a wonderful relationship and he knows my situation. (p. 311)

As well, a former researcher diagnosed with dementia noted that with the help of a former colleague, she was able to do a research project on what it is like to live with dementia. She noted that the former colleague

> came back into my life to help me make a new career, making scrambled eggs out of broken ones. Our friendship expanded into a collaboration. I could never imagine that my last research project would be a study of my own disease. (p. 311)

Can people diagnosed with dementia make new friends?

It is one thing to value and maintain the relationships one has with long-time friends, but it is quite another for a person with AD to make new friends once he or she has been diagnosed. Given that people diagnosed with AD or another type of dementia have dysfunctional explicit memory systems, especially those involved with recall, is it even possible for such people to make new friends? After all, if people have "memory loss," how could it be possible to make new friends if one cannot remember having met someone before? It usually takes a number of mutually satisfying interactions with someone before we call him or her a "friend," and one would have to be able to make memories about a new person in order to treat that person as being familiar rather than as a stranger.

There is an abundant professional literature that reveals the ability of people diagnosed to make new friends and enjoy warm, mutually caring relationships. In one study (Sabat & Lee, 2012), people in the moderate stage of dementia who attended a day center engaged in a number of mutually desired, independently initiated, supportive social relationships with people whom they met for the first time at the day center. Mrs. E expressed empathy and showed patience and understanding for Mrs. M and helped her to save face in what were potentially embarrassing situations. The same two women revealed their shared warmth in their choosing to have the experience of mutual company. Mrs. M asked Mrs. E to join her for a prayer group meeting. Mrs. E replied that, not being religious, she was not keen on attending. Mrs. M then went to the meeting. A few minutes later, after Mrs. M had chosen a seat and was settled there, Mrs. E entered the room where the meeting was being held and sat down in an empty seat next to Mrs. M even though there were many other empty seats in the room. Having Mrs. M's company was important to Mrs. E even though the two women did not share similar attitudes toward religion.

The number of participants at the previously discussed adult day center varies between approximately 20 and 30 per day (Sabat & Lee, 2012). Some people gravitate toward one another and seem always to sit together at a particular lunch table or during group activities. Mrs. E, Mrs. D, Mrs. M, and Mr. F always sat together at what became "their" table. Mrs. E commented that she loved the fact that Mr. F sat at the table with them. Mr. F had been looking at a magazine at that moment, but he heard the comment and looked at Mrs. E, who went on to talk about how, when she was 19-years old, she married a man who was in the military. Mr. F heard this and shouted out, "Was it worth it?" The group burst out in laughter. Warm interpersonal relationships are often characterized by good-natured teasing when the people involved feel close connections with one another. None of the people at the table knew any of the others before coming to the day center. Each of the people had been diagnosed with dementia in the moderate stage. Thus, even though they had memory problems severe enough to meet the diagnostic criterion for dementia, they were able to create new, durable memories of the other individuals, thereby allowing for a warm, friendly connection to develop and remain strong among them.

For this to happen, each person in the group had to possess healthy brain systems involved in "social cognition," which is defined as "cognitive abilities that enable us to make sense of our social world and to interact effectively with others. . . . Social stimuli include the self, other individuals, and social situations . . . [that] are personally relevant and mutable" (Washburn, Sands, & Walton, 2003, p. 203). Specifically, social cognition involves the processing of people's faces and facial expressions, their voices, and their posture; making judgments about others' personalities and motives; predicting their likely behavior; and planning one's own interactions with others (Adolphs, 2005). Social cognition, then, requires the use of intact sensory and perceptual functions, executive function, language and communicative skills in a variety of situations, and emotion. Additional cognitive abilities involved in social cognition include the ability to focus one's attention, the ability to perceive tones of voice and distinguish between teasing and insulting statements, perception of facial expressions, humor, working (short-term) memory, and long-term memory. Therefore, whatever memory dysfunctions are sufficient to warrant a diagnosis of dementia of whatever kind, including the Alzheimer's type, still do not prevent people from learning to make new friends of people who originally were strangers to them and to value the caring presence, the mutual acceptance, and the evident warmth of such people in their lives.

This experience is especially clear in the words of people who, while still living at home, attend a support group called Friends for Life in the United Kingdom (Ward et al., 2011). One member of the group commented, "I've really looked forward to coming to them (group meetings) and we can openly, without being ashamed, if that's another word that. . . . Be ashamed of what you're talking about, you're among friends" (p. 296). Among the reasons the members enjoy each other's company is that they can talk about dementia and what it means to them, as demonstrated by the comments of two members: "And it's not brushed under the carpet as my mam would say, you've heard that saying, haven't you?" To which the other member responded, "It's not brushed under the carpet, it's open and it's anything, don't be frightened of it" (p. 297). Sharing their experiences and enjoying the trust and safety of being together is clearly as important to people diagnosed just as it was in decades of adult life before the diagnosis, as it is to people of all ages. This is another of Kitwood's (1998) indicators of relative well-being—the acceptance of others, the appreciation of feeling safe among and trusted by others. It is clear that people who attend the Friends for Life meetings engage each other socially, empathize with one another, and provide support to and receive it from other group members, even though they have been diagnosed with AD or other types of dementia. What about people who are diagnosed but who live in nursing homes or long-term care residences?

Can people with dementia living in nursing homes have caring relationships with other residents? What challenges exist regarding life in long-term care?

Yes, but the types of relationships that develop among people diagnosed and living in nursing homes are very important to understand, especially given the social context in which the residents live. For example, compared with the life they lived for many decades as adults, they are now tremendously limited by the fact that they are not free to come and go as they please, may be restricted to living in a secure area such as a special "dementia unit" or "memory unit" within a larger building, and may be limited further by the inability to ambulate independently and the lack of control over what they do with their time (Saunders et al., 2011). This is a social world that can feel alien to say the least, and institutional care settings frequently have been found to be settings in which residents are socially isolated a great deal of the time (Ice, 2002). Given the kinds of restrictions that exist, it is perhaps not at all surprising that the level of agitation among residents diagnosed with dementia was found to be greater when they had fewer and fewer outside social contacts with friends and family not living in the nursing home (Cohen-Mansfield & Marx, 1992). Likewise, Kutner et al. (2000) found a connection between friendship and the lack of agitated behavior among 59 residents of a dementia care unit.

A brief thought experiment may be instructive here. Imagine yourself living in such an environment and having a dysfunctional explicit memory system—that is, you cannot recall why you are where you are, cannot recall how long you have been living there or how long it has been since you have seen a loved one or a friend, and you feel as though it has been forever since you saw someone whom you love and who loves you. You are told when to get up in the morning, when to bathe, when to eat, where to sit in the dining room, when to take medications whose names you do not recall nor do you recall the reason why you are taking them, and when to go to sleep. You cannot change the channel on the television that is hanging from the wall, cannot turn it off, and cannot lower or raise the volume by yourself. Perhaps you have nothing to do that is of interest to you and nowhere to go other than for a walk in the hallways or to your room. Perhaps you feel lonely, afraid, and you cannot leave even though there is nothing you would love more because you do not like being where you are. Perhaps "agitation" is the word that the staff uses to describe your actions because you are not at peace and are showing it very clearly. Would feeling a lack of inner peace under these circumstances be terribly odd? Perhaps it would be precisely how one might rightly feel. And perhaps that is why, when there is an increase in frequency of visits from family and from friends, your level of "agitation" decreases.

The fact that visits from friends and loved ones matter to people with AD or other types of dementia living in long-term care means that such people are able to value the presence of loved ones in their life, that they are able to experience and enjoy the feeling of being cared about, of being loved, and of being able to love and care about others. Imagine wanting to love and be loved and having no appropriate "targets" for those feelings, all the while knowing that those very "targets" are elsewhere. Would you not want to be with those "targets" wherever they are rather than living in the "secure dementia unit"?

If we understand "agitation" to be the way it looks to nursing home staff when people diagnosed with AD or another type of dementia are experiencing the previously discussed feelings, then we have to acknowledge that those "agitated" people have the capacity and ability to give and receive expressions of good will, to appreciate and yearn for those feelings, and to have the capacity to understand the anguish of others and provide comfort to them. It may be that such people have difficulties with spoken language due to brain damage and the resulting word-finding problems and problems speaking in syntactically correct ways, but they still may be able to express a great deal that is important among human beings.

In a series of studies (Kontos, 2004, 2005, 2012), people with AD in the moderate to severe stage and living in a long-term care home were observed to express empathy and social etiquette through their actions and words in everyday naturally occurring situations. One resident clearly showed empathy by responding with a gentle touch to another resident who was acting in an agitated way and also by providing a non-anxious presence while looking at and listening to a resident who was acting in ways that signaled being upset. Kontos (2012) provides a poignant example:

> Bertha was extremely agitated. She walked into the living room and sat down next to Ethel who was sleeping. Bertha's cries woke up Ethel, who watched her for a moment and then turned to get the attention of a personal support worker (PSW) who was attending to another resident. Ethel pointed to Bertha's shaking leg and said, "Oye, look at the leg running. She is sick." Ethel paused to hear what Bertha was saying; with a distressed look on her face she said to the PSW, "She is crying, 'oye mamma'." The PSW told Ethel not to worry and that Bertha would calm down. Ethel asked, "Is she in pain?" and the PSW assured her that she was not. Ethel, now with tears in her eyes, said, "Maybe she is hungry?" The PSW told her that Bertha is probably a little frightened. Ethel immediately put her hand on Bertha's knee and leaned close to her body, looking at her face. Bertha's cries quieted to a gentle moan. Ethel sat with her for most of the afternoon, eventually falling asleep with her hand still on Bertha's knee. Bertha too had fallen asleep. (p. 335)

Although living in a long-term care home and diagnosed with AD in the moderate to severe stage, Ethel recognized and understood the feelings of hunger and/or pain, empathized with Bertha, and provided a gentle, non-anxious presence, touching and comforting Bertha and thereby helped Bertha to feel calm and relax. Empathizing with and caring for another human being are attributes that are held in great esteem, being that they are fundamental to civility and kindness. For Ethel, who has AD, to respond as she did tells us a great deal about what AD means and does not mean. Clearly, no matter what dysfunctions she experienced in the areas of explicit memory, calculation, organization of movement, planning, and language, Ethel was still able to act in a way that exemplifies deeply valued qualities in human beings. In other words, AD did not take away from Ethel the ability to show empathy, kindness, concern, and gentility toward another person. And if she can feel the discomfort of another person's fright or pain or hunger, she can also feel those things in herself and can be hurt by the unkindness of others. As well, Ethel can also benefit greatly from the kindness, love, and attention of others. Finally, it is clear that Bertha was able to regain a feeling of calm not with pharmacological intervention but, rather, by Ethel's personal, empathetic presence.

The mere attention of another person can be of great value in transforming a moment into something special. Kontos (2012) notes,

> Bertha and Anna were seated across from one another in the lounge. Suddenly, their eyes met and Anna smiled. Anna's smile triggered a smile in Bertha, making her resonate with animation. The sudden appearance of a smile on Bertha's face . . . transformed her usual expressionless face. Bertha's smile seemed to reanimate Anna's fading smile. Several moments ensued of linked smiles back and forth. (p. 337)

Without uttering a single word, the two women exchanged warm attention and created what Pringle (2003) described as enhancing the quality of the moment. Interestingly, in this article, Pringle was talking about how professionals such as nurses could work to enhance the quality of the moment, but in this case, it was two long-term care residents diagnosed with AD who, by their own actions, accomplished this important deed.

A final example from Kontos's 2012 study is especially meaningful for a variety of reasons that I discuss following a recounting of the interpersonal interaction itself:

> Edna was in a terrible state of agitation. She walked along the hallways calling out for her son Ernie. As she passed the living room she saw Florence sleeping on the sofa. She immediately sat down next to her and placed her hand on Florence's forearm. Florence jolted slightly as she opened her eyes. Edna quickly said to her, "I want to know when I'm going home. I don't know anyone here." Florence took her free hand and placed it on top of Edna's hand, which was still on Florence's forearm, and replied in a reassuring tone, "You know me." Still agitated, Edna said, "I'm completely lost," holding her hands out in despair. Still very calm, Florence replied, "I've been there" pushing her hands in a swiftly downward motion with a sharp flick of the wrists as if to say, "don't worry about it." (p. 339)

In this interchange, Edna was clearly upset, frightened, feeling lost, and terribly vulnerable. Florence understood what Edna was feeling and first called Edna's attention, in a non-anxious way, to the fact that Edna was not without a person she knows—for there was Florence whom she knows ("You know me"). When Florence said that she felt lost, Florence empathized with her and tried to communicate that that feeling will pass and there is nothing to worry about. Florence was providing a safe space for Edna; was being calm, caring, and empathetic; and was doing what a true friend, or at least a caring human being, would do even though she was diagnosed with AD in the moderate to severe stage. In order for Florence to have responded as she did to Edna, she had to have been able to understand not only the words that Edna spoke but also the emotional tone and meaning of what Edna said. In

addition, she had to have been in possession of memory functions that allowed her to know that Edna knew her and that
she knew Edna. This would not be possible if Florence had a
condition called "memory loss." It is also fascinating to consider that Florence may not have been able to state correctly
the day of the week, the month, the year, the season, and the
like, but all that had nothing to do with her ability to act in a
positive, caring, empathetic way. She knew how to make the
moment better for Edna just the same.

If Florence possesses the ability to help ease another's
anguish, it stands to reason that she would be able to appreciate being treated in the same way if she were experiencing
anguish herself. Furthermore, we see demonstrated vividly in
Anna, Bertha, and Ethel the reality that having a diagnosis of
AD and living in a long-term care home does not mean that a
person is bereft of the ability to care about others' well-being,
the ability to recognize and appreciate the feelings of others,
and the ability to soothe someone when he or she is upset. In
other words, having this diagnosis does not mean that a person
is "demented," and the person should not be spoken about,
thought of, or treated as if he or she were. Indeed, feelings
and displays of empathy have been thought of as being connected intimately to "caring imagination" (Hamington, 2004).
In order to empathize with another person, one must be able to
imagine how one would feel if one were in the other person's
position. If one had no mind, one would not be able to imagine anything at all. Indeed, it may be worth considering that
the way medical professionals define "cognition," or thinking,
needs serious revision. I say this because cognition is typically
"measured" by neuropsychological tests, but these tests do not
examine the entire family of abilities that people use and display in the everyday social world. Although they have their
appropriate uses, the tests are, in a very real way, artificial and
limited. They may be used as objective outcome measures to
assess the efficacy of drugs, but that does not mean that they
tell us the whole story about a person's ability to think and

feel and react in the natural social world. Thus, a dysfunction in cognition as measured by tests does not mean a complete dysfunction regarding empathy and imagination as they are demonstrated in natural interpersonal interactions.

All this, in turn, means that a diagnosis of dementia of the Alzheimer's type in the moderate to severe stage does not necessarily leave a person living in long-term care bereft of the ability to feel for others, to care about others, to benefit from being cared about and empathized with, to need, and to thrive in the presence of supportive caring others.

Is this true for everyone diagnosed with Alzheimer's disease or another dementia and living in long-term care?

It is impossible to say that Anna, Bertha, and Ethel are representative of every person who shares their diagnosis and living arrangement. There have not been nearly enough studies of people living in long-term care homes by researchers who are willing and able to take the great amount of time and care necessary to observe and come to know residents diagnosed. Researchers must be able to become part of the residential community and make their own observations of people on a day-to-day basis rather than obtaining "snapshots" of interactions on a few particular days.

It is relevant also to raise the question, Does everyone who is *not* diagnosed and *not* living in long-term care display sensitivity, empathy, and care as did the women with AD? It seems safe to say that people are not all equally sensitive, empathetic, and caring, so why should we expect, even theoretically, everyone diagnosed to possess these qualities equally? Perhaps the more important question is, Can a person diagnosed with AD or another type of dementia in the moderate to severe stages and who can no longer live independently or be taken care of at home by family *remain able* to be sensitive, caring, empathetic toward others? If this is the question, the answer is "yes."

Even if this is not true of everyone, it would seem only fair to give people diagnosed the benefit of the doubt and assume that they have these abilities to one or another degree rather than assume that they do not. Assuming that other people so diagnosed possess these abilities to some degree would be based on observations such as those reported here. Assuming that people diagnosed do not have these abilities would be based on negative stereotypes and the performance of those diagnosed on standard neuropsychological tests that, as discussed previously, have little to nothing to do with the abilities in question as they are demonstrated in the natural, everyday social world. What is needed is the opportunity to observe interpersonal interactions that could reveal these qualities in people.

Why can't we just interview long-term care home staff members and hear what they say about people diagnosed?

Although it may be possible in principle to do this, long-term care staff members' perceptions of residents' friendships were not supported by observations made by independent researchers who spent 6 months at a particular long-term care home (de Medeiros et al., 2011). For example, although the staff identified four men who sat at what the staff called "the men's table" as being friends and said that conversations were the basis of those friendships, direct observations of these men revealed few verbal and nonverbal interactions among them. By contrast, one of the men who was not seated at the "men's table," Carl, had multiple conversations with a woman, Lucy, and both named the other as being a friend during individual interviews, even though the staff did not identify these two people as being friends.

Of course, the ability of independent researchers to observe and interview residents is an important factor here because staff members have a great deal of responsibility and need to attend to a variety of matters concerning the residents, leaving them far less time to make detailed observations of, much less interview, residents. Therefore, it may be questionable to use staff members' reports alone to learn about the kinds of relationships that exist among residents. What is needed is the detailed qualitative understanding of the depth of those relationships, many of which are revealed in relatively brief but very meaningful daily encounters such as revealed in Kontos's research and that of de Medeiros et al. described herein.

It is clear, I think, that people diagnosed with AD or another type of dementia retain a number of psychological/emotional and cognitive strengths. In order for the person diagnosed to flourish, those strengths must be noticed, appreciated, respected, and encouraged by healthy others, be they family care partners or professionals. When the person diagnosed can live to his or her full potential, care partners of all kinds can do the same and everyone benefits. Important aspects of this process include the resilience of the person diagnosed and that of his or her care partners, as well as the strengthening of the selfhood of all concerned. These key factors are addressed in Chapter 5.

5

RESILIENCE, SELFHOOD, AND CREATIVITY

Kate Swaffer is co-founder and co-chair of Dementia Alliance International, chair of the Alzheimer's Australia Dementia Advisory Committee, and speaks internationally to educate people about dementia and enlightened care of people diagnosed. In 2015, she was among the finalists in the Australian of the Year Awards and received the Dementia Leader of the Year Award. All this would be noteworthy under any circumstances, but it is perhaps even more remarkable because in 2008 she was diagnosed with younger onset dementia, a diagnosis reconfirmed in 2009. She was 49 years old. Her compelling book *What the Hell Happened to My Brain?* was published in 2016. In one of her many articles, she wrote, "Dementia is the only disease or condition and the only terminal illness that I know of where patients are told to go home and give up their pre-diagnosis lives, rather than to 'fight for their lives'" (Swaffer, 2015, p. 3). Kate is a wonderfully humane human being who has learned, and continues to learn, to live well with dementia. The same can be said about Christine Bryden, who was diagnosed with dementia at the age of 46 years in 1995 when she was a single mother of three children. Since then, she has written three books and has been *Dancing with Dementia*, the title of one of her books, while working to challenge the negative stereotypes of people with dementia and to help create supportive environments for people diagnosed. Since her diagnosis, in addition to writing and speaking at conferences, she met and married Paul Bryden. Christine had to tell Paul about her diagnosis early in their relationship, and when she did, with understandable trepidation, he responded immediately by saying something like "We can work with that." One might say that Kate and Christine are tremendously resilient, given their diagnoses and what they have done with their lives since then, but that really begs the question, What is resilience and how does a person become resilient?

What is resilience and how does one become resilient?

Although we can think of a person as being resilient, there is still the question of how one becomes resilient. After all, it is great to be resilient, but it is unlikely that some people are simply born that way and others are not and that is the end of the story. Therefore, contemporary researchers such as Windle (2012) suggest that resilience is a process whereby one deals with or adapts to some kind of trauma by using factors within oneself, one's life, or in the environment to cope with or recover from that trauma. Windle notes, "This definition acknowledges key features of resilience: (1) the encounter with adversity such as ill health, (2) the ability to resist, manage, and adapt to adversity (drawing on resources), and (3) the maintenance of good mental health" (p. 159). Among the factors possibly connected to resilience in later life are supportive social networks and spiritual support (Yee-Melichar, 2011). Researchers are examining the roles of optimism and problem solving as well (Lavretsky, 2014; Smith & Hayslip, 2012). Clearly, Kate Swaffer and Christine Bryden exemplify the three features of resilience previously mentioned, but it is also clear that very important factors, or resources, in their lives include the patience and loving support of their husbands and the presence of strong supportive social networks. One way that they have been able to "resist, manage, and adapt" to the adversity that dementia involves is by having a mission in life: to educate people about the experience of dementia, the strengths still possessed by people diagnosed, how to support and build upon those strengths, as well as how to reduce the occurrence of malignant social psychology in their lives and the lives of others diagnosed. Each woman has a cause that is bigger than herself, which is one way to live a fulfilling life irrespective of a diagnosis of dementia of any kind. The great value of such a "mission" was clear as well in my own work (Sabat, 2001, 2003), wherein I engaged people diagnosed with Alzheimer's disease (AD) as my teachers who could speak with authority so that others might learn what it is like to have AD. Mrs. B, Dr. B's wife, noted that this work gave great meaning to the last 9 months of his life.

Is there any research on resiliency and people with Alzheimer's disease or other types of dementia?

There is not a great deal of this type of research, but what does exist is certainly thought-provoking. For example, Harris (2016) interviewed 20 people between ages 54 and 84 years who were diagnosed with early stage dementia and interviewed their care partners as well. Of these, she focused on 10 people—5 who demonstrated resilience and 5 who did not. The difference depended on whether or not the person (1) had faced and overcome adversity or was facing adversity presently and (2) was doing "okay" as defined by appropriate healthy functioning and engaging life in the face of dementia.

The characteristics of people in each group were strikingly different in very important ways. People who were doing "okay" had accepted their diagnosis and decided to do the best they could with their lives, whereas those who were not doing "okay" did not accept the diagnosis and felt that they might as well give up. Those who were doing "okay" maintained a positive, optimistic attitude, not allowing what goes wrong to fester within them, whereas those who were not doing "okay" became angry with themselves in reaction to things going amiss. The resilient people remained engaged with others in relationships involving mutual giving and receiving, whereas those who were not resilient refrained from going out in public for fear of embarrassing themselves and being spoken about negatively by others.

The presence of supportive family and friends had a great effect on the degree to which people diagnosed displayed resilience. Care partners of those who were resilient were more patient than before, attended closely to what their loved one said, and did not automatically underestimate their loved one's ability. They strived to help their loved one maintain as much independence as possible, attended to his or her opinions about sundry matters, and involved their loved one in decision-making tasks. Recall the interaction between Mrs. B and Dr. B when she would pick him up at the adult day center: He would always ask, "Okay, what are we doing?" and she would always respond, "What would you like to do?" because she wanted him to know that she was aware of and respected the fact that he had desires and she believed that he ought to be actively involved in deciding what they would do together. Conversely, the care partners of those who did not display resilience were angry or resentful about "the bad dream" they were living, felt robbed of their lives, did not recognize a relationship to exist between themselves and their loved ones, believed they had to take charge of everything, and did not respect their loved one's intelligence. For example, just as I was beginning a presentation to a group of care partners, one spousal care partner shouted, "They don't know anything anymore" about people diagnosed.

In terms of connections to the wider social community, resilient people sought out and received help from supportive services, such as from health care providers and others; did volunteer work; were engaged with the Alzheimer's Association; and enjoyed regular exercise. Conversely, those who were not resilient were socially isolated and had few connections with heath care providers and other professionals. In a nutshell, people who were resilient were still viewed as whole persons by their care partners and were still actively engaged in life, whereas the opposite was true for people who were not resilient.

These findings provide valuable information for everyone, really, not just those of us who are living with the effects of AD or another type of dementia. Indeed, there is a great truth in the idea that what people can do to help those diagnosed to live fulfilling lives is very similar to what each of us can do to help people who are not diagnosed, including ourselves, to live good lives. But more to the present point,

What does Harris's research mean specifically for helping people diagnosed?

In Harris's (2016) study, the first characteristic that differentiated people with dementia who were doing okay from those who were not was that the former had accepted their condition, whereas those who were not doing okay had not and had decided that they may as well give up. Therefore, it is important for care partners and those diagnosed to accept the diagnosis and to decide to work together to make the best of the moments that remain to them.

A wonderful example of acceptance not related to dementia but worthy of consideration nonetheless was displayed by the great Hall of Fame baseball player Roy Campanella, who, while he was still an active player on the Brooklyn Dodgers, was in an automobile accident that left him quadriplegic. In his book *The Boys of Summer*, Roger Kahn (1971) described a poignant interaction he had with Campanella years after the accident—after Roy's wife separated from him and died 3 years later, and after he was remarried to Roxie Doles, who loved him deeply. In conversing with Kahn, Campanella, seated in his wheelchair, recounted that after he was diagnosed with fractures of the fifth and sixth cervical vertebrae and a compressed spinal cord, his physician, Howard Rusk, told him, "You may get to walk again and you may not. If you don't, you'll have to learn to live with it." Kahn wrote,

> Very softly, Campanella said, "I think I've learned how … I've accepted the chair. … My family has accepted it. My wife has made a wonderful home. I'm not wanting many things. Sure, I'd love to walk. Sure I would. But I'm not gonna worry myself to death because I can't. I've accepted the chair and I've accepted my life." He pushed the lever and the wheelchair started off bearing the broken body and leaving me, and perhaps Roxie Campanella as well, to marvel at the vaulting human spirit, imprisoned yet free, in the noble wreckage of the athlete, in the dazzling palace of the man. (p. 341)

Although Campanella's injury did not affect his cognitive abilities, the damage was permanent and irreversible, and he and his family responded by choosing the path of acceptance and lived without anger, recrimination, or regret. They made their lives as worthy of living as they could and found as much joy together as they could in the face of an incurable trauma.

Christine and Paul Bryden and Kate Swaffer and her husband, Peter, have faced dementia together precisely as Roxie and Roy Campanella faced his paralysis, and their level of acceptance has allowed all of them to do great good with their days, even in the presence of the often staggering and unremitting difficulties that dementia entails. In the process, they have been optimistic, drawing on the long-time strengths of the person diagnosed, and this has led both women to view their condition as an opportunity to work on behalf of others who share their diagnosis. It is just as important, however, to recognize that even when people can accept their condition gracefully, find a reserve of optimism and the will to go on and do all they can within the new limits that they experience due to brain damage, they also require time and the feeling of safety to grieve. This applies to the person diagnosed as well as to his or her care partners.

Does resilience involve grieving as well?

Grieving one's losses is as much a part of life as is exulting in and celebrating one's achievements. As we learn from Ecclesiastes, "There is a time to weep and a time to laugh, a time to mourn and a time to dance." When Kate Swaffer asks, "What the hell happened to my brain?" she is not in a celebratory mood, and she, as does each of us, needs to be able to grieve her losses without filling all her moments with grief. That is one of the delicate, nuanced balances that can be appreciated as being one goal of living with AD and other forms of dementia. Indeed, the ability to grieve, to mourn, the loss of cherished abilities ought to be added to the list of "indicators of relative well-being" that Kitwood (1998) articulated. Grief is surely an appropriate response to such situations, but at times even well-intentioned care partners can misunderstand expressions of grief.

For example, Mrs. L was the primary care partner for her mother, who was diagnosed with AD and living with Mrs. L and her husband. Mrs. L was very upset because her mother spent a great deal of time at home crying even though there was no obvious provocation. Accordingly, she interpreted her mother's crying as "irrational" and caused by AD. Mrs. L's brother lived in the area and spent a good amount of time with his mother. When Mrs. L's mother was with her son, she did not cry at all, and Mrs. L said that "she behaved herself" at those times. Upon questioning Mrs. L further, I learned that over the course of many decades Mrs. L's mother was much more open emotionally with Mrs. L than with her son. Apparently, the diagnosis of AD had not changed that dynamic in their relationship. Mrs. L's mother was still far more open emotionally with her daughter than she was with her son and thus did not cry when she was with her son. At this point, Mrs. L understood clearly that her role was not so much to stop her mother from crying, from grieving, but rather to be the person with whom her mother could safely, openly, fully express her justifiable grief (Sabat, 2001). It is simultaneously clear from the research literature that one way to achieve that nuanced balance between grief and "dancing with dementia," as Christine Bryden called her experience, is to have the support of family and friends.

How can family and friends contribute to resilience?

Encouraging people with dementia and their families to make their diagnoses known to close friends is also important to the process of resilience, just as is communicating to close friends that the person diagnosed needs to feel safe—safe from negative stereotyping, for example. In this way, people close to the person diagnosed know that they have a very important role to play in their friend's life. This role would also involve educating others about malignant social psychology and how it can diminish the self-worth of people diagnosed. Friends can thereby help to erase those actions from the social world they share with people diagnosed and, in turn, communicate what they have learned to others so as to change, gradually, the public perception of dementia. As well, friends can help by focusing on the diagnosed person's strengths and keeping their friendships alive by accepting the person diagnosed as they always did in the past and not withdrawing from their friend's life.

Can support groups aid the process of resilience?

For many people, support groups can be very helpful. One example is Bill and his wife Kathleen, who were among Lisa Snyder's (2009) subjects in her book, *Speaking Our Minds*. The couple agreed to participate in an 8-week support group meant to educate couples about living with AD. Bill said,

I jumped at the opportunity. I had been diagnosed for two years but I had never known or even seen another patient! I was a bit nervous, but I looked forward to meeting new friends that I could relate to. When we first glanced at the group, I thought we were in the wrong room because everyone else was at least 10 or 20 years older than us. But that distinction began to melt away when we found that we were all in the same boat and in that sense, all the same age. (p. 48)

This very stark situation is just one of many confronted by people who are diagnosed with young-onset dementia. Bill's experience of the group is tremendously instructive, as he said,

The real value of the group was that we were getting to know others—both patients and caregivers. I was also made aware of the different courses the disease takes ... I wasn't able to find my words, but others chattered along without a care. Sometimes they said the same thing over and over! (p. 48)

Being able to share experiences including hopes, sadness, frustrations, and laughter with others is extremely important for many people whether or not they have been diagnosed with AD or another type of dementia. There can be solace in feeling understood by another person after you have spoken about something important to you, in being accepted by others unconditionally. It is reasonable to assume that this need remains for people even after having been diagnosed. The fact that during the 2 years since he was diagnosed Bill had not met another person with the same diagnosis reflected a type of social isolation in his life.

Through this group, Bill came to feel part of a larger community of people diagnosed and wanted to have more such contact after the 8-week session ended: "I want a support group for us—for patients ... I cannot understand why there are so many support groups for caregivers and none for the afflicted!" (Snyder, 2009, p. 49). As a result, the San Diego chapter of the Alzheimer's Association created a program called "The Morning Out Club," and Lisa Snyder began developing a regular support group for people diagnosed. In so doing, she displayed how deeply she valued and respected Bill's point of view, his intelligence, and his ability to articulate a need that, as it turned out, he was hardly alone in feeling. The support group for people with AD became a reality as a result of Lisa's work and the cooperation of many others at the Shiley–Marcos Alzheimer's Research Center at the University of California at San Diego, and it turned out to be extremely important for Bill as well as for the other group members. One reason why Bill enjoyed the group meetings so much was that they provided him with something different in a day-to-day life that had become routine to the point of being troublesome due its lack of varied and enlivening experiences. He said that he loved the group, that "It's joyous. It can't be bottled" (p. 54).

The group was a way for Bill to share his thoughts, hopes, his very being, with others. For example, he had written poems for his wife, Kathleen, during their years of marriage, and parts of some of his poems were read at the end of each support group meeting. By this time, Bill had lost a great deal of his fluency in speaking and in finding the words that would capture his thoughts. This was especially difficult because he was extremely verbal in the past, having been a magazine editor for the Foreign Service Division of the US Information Agency. He was an artist with words and linguistic expression; writing was his paintbrush and the blank page his canvas. As he grieved the loss of the cherished ability that he enjoyed so much for so long, his voice was still heard by having his poetry read at the support group meetings. In this way, the other group members, as well as the group leader, came to know and appreciate Bill in a deeply meaningful way. His poems reflected the person Bill had always been, and that aspect of his being remained alive even though AD had now interfered with his ability to manifest it via speaking in the moment. The beauty of those moments in the support group meetings was that he could still shine, and his words and thoughts helped to make good moments for the other group members as well as for him.

Not only did Bill's comment lead to the development of the support group but he indicated as well that he had still another purpose, greater than himself, that he wanted to fulfill: "As difficult as it is for me to read and write anymore or to talk about myself, I think it is important therapy for me and a help to others to know what I am experiencing" (Snyder, 2009, p. 36). The idea of doing something to help others is a type of sophisticated thinking and goal setting that deserves appreciation and admiration when displayed by any of us, really, as well as by someone diagnosed with AD. Once again, we learn that the brain damage that causes a diagnosis of dementia of the Alzheimer's type does not necessarily erase the ability to consider the well-being of others and how one might contribute to the greater good of the community. This is yet another example of resilience demonstrated by a person diagnosed with AD.

As we grow from being children to adults, we increasingly appreciate the degree to which we are interdependent, how much we truly do need one another as we seek to experience lives worth living. We learn also that it is possible to grow in the face of traumatic experiences and that, in some cases, our greatest leaps in personal growth occur when we are confronted with challenges of great magnitude, when we experience trauma. This is true with dementia just as it is with other sorts of trauma we may face, and approaching dementia with this optimistic attitude truly does make a difference for the better in the lives of persons diagnosed and those of the people around them. This begs us to ask whether people can grow after they are diagnosed.

Is it possible for people to grow after they have been diagnosed?

More than 20 years ago, Kitwood's (1995) interviews with health care professionals revealed dozens of instances of people living with dementia who had experienced changes for the good in their lives. For example, for some there was increased assertiveness in the degree of trust toward others, enhanced warmth and affection, as well as acceptance of losses and limitations. Relatively recently, research in Japan (Fukushima et al., 2005) included reports by family care partners indicating that loved ones diagnosed displayed a number of positive changes in the aftermath of struggling with the losses they experienced due to brain damage. People diagnosed came to accept the diagnosis, displayed more relaxed demeanors than they had previously, developed a greater appreciation of the present moments of their lives than they had evidenced in previous years, and were more sensitive to and grateful for the contributions that other people made to their lives. Snyder (2009) reported similar positive changes in Bill, who came to enjoy going for walks with his wife and took great delight, as never before, in the vibrant beauty of nature.

Even more recently, Wolverson and Patterson (2016) reported a study of nine people and their experience of positive and meaningful changes in their lives while living with dementia. When interviewed about their experiences, people diagnosed reported experiencing a kind of evolution in their approaches to life in that, more than ever before, they were motivated to find positive experiences, especially given the fleeting nature of time. Not wanting to waste time on things about which they were powerless to change (similar to what Roy Campanella said about his paralysis) was one of the most profound changes for the better that was reported. Other interviewees reported feeling deeper compassion than they had before living with dementia. They also reported feeling more attentive to and appreciative of the present than they had before. Thus, some people reported that they no longer procrastinated because they did not know what tomorrow would bring.

All this is not meant to convey that there is something called "successful" living with dementia because that would imply by definition that there was the possibility of "unsuccessful" living with dementia or "failure" at doing so. There has been much discussion and more than one book published in recent years about "successful aging." I do not believe that this is a helpful way to think about life. After all, we do not talk about "successful" childhood, "successful" adolescence, "successful" young adulthood, or "successful" midlife, so there is no logical reason to apply this descriptor to aging or to living with traumatic experiences or with dementia. There are simply many different ways of coping, of living, and there are as many different ways of doing so with dementia as there are of living life in general.

The important point here, I think, is that some people have demonstrated through their words and deeds that it is possible to continue to live and grow and to appreciate life even after having been diagnosed. As well, they show that dementia is not necessarily some kind of living death, and that it is a great challenge to each of us to find what Lincoln called "the better angels of our nature" so that we, as human beings, can help one another as best we can through experiences such as living with dementia. Knowing life with dementia does not have to be "a living death" or a "long goodbye" and that it is still possible to make good moments with and for one another is potentially empowering for each of us.

From the work of both Harris and Snyder, we learned that among the ways to promote optimism and hope in people diagnosed is to identify a person's lifelong strengths and history of adaptation and coping styles and to keep in mind that the period of the person's life characterized by the diagnosis of dementia is but another chapter after many others. A helpful way to accomplish this is to examine aspects of the person's selfhood. This has been a topic of much discussion in part because it has been alleged in more than one arena that AD entails a "loss of self" (Cohen & Eisdorfer, 2002). We should not take this at face value, however. As it is for everyone, self-hood is a complex issue for people with dementia. So we must step back and ask whether there is a loss of selfhood in those with dementia.

Is there a loss of selfhood in people with dementia?

This is not the place to explore the various proposals offered regarding the nature of the self, for philosophers and scientists have pondered it for centuries. I surely do not have the answers. But the question of how one's self is affected by dementia is important and is importantly connected to resilience and the question of how can we enhance optimism and hope while reducing despair in people diagnosed. After all, it is much more difficult to go on living one's life if one feels that there is a complete break between "who I was before dementia" and "who I am now." As much as possible, we must help people diagnosed to appreciate the continuity in themselves from before to after the diagnosis. To do this, we must be attentive to their selfhood.

Social constructionist theory, advanced in the 20th century by Rom Harré (1983, 1991) and applied to people with AD (Sabat, 2001; Sabat & Harré, 1992, 1994), can be used as a tool to help us understand how dementia does or does not affect a person's selfhood. In this way of thinking, the self has three different aspects called Self 1, Self 2, and Self 3. Let us examine them in order.

Self 1 is the experience of oneself as an individual who is one and the same person from moment to moment. This stands in contrast to a person who has multiple personality disorder, in which he or she can claim to be a fundamentally different person from moment to moment. Self 1 is expressed through the use of personal pronouns such as "I," "me," "my," "we" (you and I), and "us" (you and me). So if a person said, "I don't even know my name," the use of "I" and "my" indicates the presence of Self 1—an individual who is experiencing the inability to recall his or her name. Self 1 can be expressed also by pointing to oneself if one cannot speak. AD and other types of dementia do not necessarily erase this aspect of selfhood even in the severe stages.

Self 2 is the aspect of selfhood that is composed of one's mental and physical attributes, past and present. Among one's physical attributes are one's height, skin pigmentation, eye pigmentation, facial hair or lack thereof, age, health status, a diagnosis of dementia of one or another type, and the like. Among one's mental attributes are one's beliefs (religious, spiritual, political, ethical, etc.), one's intellectual achievements (high school grad, college grad, holder of advanced degrees, and others), other proclivities such as one's ability and desire (or lack thereof) to do complicated crossword puzzles or Sudoku, one's proficiency in languages or mathematics (or lack thereof), one's sense of humor (or lack thereof), one's difficulties in finding the words one wants to use, one's memory dysfunction, and so on. Recall that when the director of the adult day center introduced Henry, a participant diagnosed with AD, to another person and said, "This is Henry. Henry was a lawyer," Henry interrupted immediately and said, "I *am* a lawyer." Henry was correct because he had a degree from law school, had not been disbarred, and being an attorney remained one of his attributes even though he was no longer practicing law. Self 2 includes positive as well as negative attributes, gains as well as losses. Another part of Self 2 is one's beliefs about one's attributes: We may take pride in some of our attributes and may be embarrassed or ashamed about others.

Dementia of any type does not erase Self 2, but we can appreciate part of the predicament of the person diagnosed by doing a brief thought experiment. Think of one attribute about which you are not happy—some habit you have, perhaps a tendency to procrastinate, or perhaps you smoke or do text messaging while driving. Whichever attribute it is, it should be something you really do not like about yourself, want to change, and perhaps have tried to change. Thus far, however, you have been unable to change it, and you feel frustrated and unhappy, perhaps even guilty, as a result. Imagine how you would feel if everyone you encountered saw you principally for that one attribute while mostly or completely ignoring a host of other valued, positive attributes you possess. In other words, you are being seen and understood by others primarily in terms of the one attribute you loathe, that you cannot stand—the one attribute that you like least about yourself. How would you feel? Would you feel embarrassed, ashamed? Would you want to avoid people because they would automatically see you as an instance of the thing(s) you like least about yourself?

Essentially, this is one of many predicaments that people diagnosed with AD and other dementias experience every day. This is why people such as Bill enjoy being in a support group that provides them with acceptance and the opportunity to be seen as human beings who possess a host of admirable, valued, Self 2 attributes. Each of us wants to be appreciated for our virtues and accepted despite our foibles. People diagnosed with dementia have lived decades of adult life in exactly this way, but now they face the challenge of being seen mostly as someone diagnosed, someone who has "memory loss" (another misunderstanding, as discussed in Chapter 4), someone who cannot speak well anymore, or someone who "used to be" an admirable person but who now is mostly, if not completely, defined by negative Self 2 attributes—someone to whom others are saying "the long goodbye."

Simultaneously, the person diagnosed can be painfully aware of the changes that have occurred in his or her long-valued Self 2 attributes and feel tormented by the changes and, hence, grieve what has been lost. Snyder's (2009) interviews with Bill reflected this strikingly in what he said with regard to a manuscript he began writing a year after he was diagnosed. For 2 years, this exceptionally articulate man wrote about what was happening to him as a result of AD, exactly while the progress of the disease was robbing him, slowly but surely, of the ability to find the words he wanted to use to convey his abundant thoughts. One day, after he could no longer write or type, he looked at the manuscript and said, "I can't believe I wrote this. . . . It ma . . . it makes . . . it makes me . . . bad, n . . . n . . . not bad . . . I can't . . . I can't . . . sad. Where . . . where did it . . . did all . . . all that (ability) go?" (p. 52). Although a person may have the upsetting Self 2 attribute of memory dysfunction that prevents him or her from recalling recent events, the memory of valued Self 2 attributes can remain quite alive and well. Also alive and well is the ability to compare those valued attributes as they existed in the past with the way they exist in the present. Another of Snyder's subjects, Jean, articulated this very well when she commented that it was not the idea of death that she found disturbing but, rather, the loss of aspects of herself (Self 2 attributes she valued) that was terribly disturbing. So someone can say, "I don't feel like myself" as a result. This is another example of the diagnosed person's ability to make meaning—to understand the meaning of circumstances and events—which is another Self 2 attribute that can remain intact even in the moderate to severe stages of dementia.

We can use this information to help the person who is living this situation. We can recognize the need and the occasion to provide sensitive consolation, and we can also recognize the need to be with the person in ways that acknowledge and respect the admirable Self 2 attributes that he or she has possessed and still possesses. To take Henry, the day center participant with a diagnosis of AD and who still is a lawyer, as an example, we can interact with him in ways that show awareness of and respect for his academic and professional achievements, even if it includes initially, and at various other times, addressing him as "counselor," for example. I have found that addressing retired university faculty members as "professor" is a very helpful way to interact. We can openly acknowledge and appreciate all the good qualities the person has and has had because those attributes still form the person's Self 2. We thereby engage the person with attention to his or her historic strengths and adaptations to significant challenges. This is what it means to inspire optimism and hope—to let the person diagnosed know clearly and concretely that we do not view him or her primarily as someone diagnosed with AD or another type of dementia. That is, we make it clear that we do not view him or her as a jumble of pathological symptoms, as an instance of someone with a disease, but, rather, as a person of value who possesses admirable attributes.

A third part of the self according to social constructionist theory is *Self 3* or, more accurately, *Selves 3*, the socially presented aspect of us. This aspect of selfhood is very vulnerable to AD or other forms of dementia. Each of us has a number of social personae—ways of being, of acting, with people—and each persona is different from the next because we have different social relationships with each of a variety of people. For example, the same person can be an authoritative teacher; a devoted, loving parent; a respectful, loving, and deferential adult child; a loving, romantic spouse; a loyal friend; a kind neighbor; a polite and loyal customer; and so on. Each of these relationships is different from the others, each has its own unique pattern of action or way of being, and the codes of conduct and behavior are different in each case to fit with the social context. So each of us has many different social selves, as it were, according to social constructionist theory.

There is another aspect of the Self 3 that is critical in relation to dementia: In order for any Self 3 persona to come into being, the cooperation of at least one other person is required. Therefore, one cannot "construct" the persona of "demanding supervisor" if one's subordinates do not recognize him or her as being their supervisor; one cannot construct the persona of "authoritative teacher" without the cooperation of one's students. We can, therefore, appreciate that any particular Self 3 persona/social self is continuously co-created in the interaction of at least two people. As discussed later, this is especially important in the lives of people diagnosed with AD or another type of dementia. First, however, let us explore another aspect of the many social personae that each of us can construct because this also is very important in connection with people diagnosed.

You might relate easily to the experience of having seen someone in only one social context, perhaps a teacher in school or a supervisor at work, and then being utterly surprised when you see the "authoritative teacher" or "demanding supervisor" acting in a silly, giddy, sing-song way when playing with his or her little child or grandchild. The surprise is a result of two important factors:

1. You experienced the teacher or supervisor in only one social context up to that point.
2. Very critically, you have created a mental storyline or narrative about that person based on this limited experience. That storyline or narrative is very limited so that what you think about how the authoritative teacher "really is" does not allow for the actions he or she engages in when playing with a child. Therefore, you do not expect that person to be capable of acting in a silly way and it is therefore a surprise, even a shock.

In my own experience, I still remember how, as an undergraduate student, I was utterly shocked when I discovered that my eloquent, rather distinguished, professor was quite knowledgeable about sports. I had created a storyline in my mind about professors and thought that they were so caught up in the life of esoteric intellectual pursuits that they would never bother paying attention to things comparatively trifling as baseball, for example.

How does all this relate to people with Alzheimer's disease or another dementia?

The social constructionist approach would lead to several conclusions. First, dementia does not result in a loss of Self 1, for as long as the person diagnosed uses first-person pronouns verbally or nonverbally (via gesture), this aspect of selfhood is intact.

Second, Self 2 is also intact because the person diagnosed always has attributes past and present. What the diagnosed person faces, however, is the possibility that others in his or her social world will focus increasingly on the dysfunctional attributes that are connected to AD/dementia and increasingly less on the attributes that he or she values dearly. Being seen principally for one's dysfunctions can create a very unhealthy and unhelpful situation for the person diagnosed, for it can create a tremendous assault on his or her feelings of self-worth. It could make someone want to avoid others, for rather good reason: literally to protect him- or herself. At the same time, this surely does not help the person's resilience.

Finally, we come to Self/Selves 3 and people with dementia. Recall that in order for a person with AD, or anyone for that matter, to construct a particular Self 3 persona, the person requires the cooperation of another person or persons. Given this situation, the person with dementia is particularly vulnerable because

- as long as healthy others focus mostly on the diagnosed person's dysfunctional Self 2 attributes due to AD and attend increasingly less to the Self 2 attributes that the person values,
- the diagnosed person will have increasingly more difficulty gaining the cooperation needed to construct a valued Self 3 persona. This means that if others see the person diagnosed as primarily defective and confused, and they develop storylines about the person that emphasize those dysfunctions, it will be difficult, if not impossible, for the person with AD or another dementia to construct a social persona other than "the burdensome, defective patient." In short order, others will come to believe that that is all the person with AD *can be*. Under

these circumstances, it is a very short step to interpreting what truly is the person's righteous indignation as being his or her irrational hostility instead—interpreting what is truly appropriate anxiety, loneliness, and trepidation as being disease-caused agitation instead, thus requiring medication rather than an understanding, soothing, non-anxious presence and active listening on the part of healthy others.

If, however, the person with dementia does receive the necessary cooperation from others, he or she will be able to construct valued, healthy Self 3 personae even when in the moderate to severe stages of AD, such as did Dr. M and Dr. B (Sabat, 2001). Dr. M, you recall, was the retired professor of sociology who had severe word-finding problems that prevented her from speaking with the exceptional ability she enjoyed since childhood. She and I would take long walks through some woods behind her home to and along a path that runs alongside the Chesapeake and Ohio Canal. She knew the area well and would lead me the whole way, as I was initially completely unfamiliar with where we were and were we were going. She was very agile and able to navigate across and through the uneven ground in the woods, whereas I, wearing dress shoes, was quite unsteady on my feet, unsure of myself. During our walks, her speech was much more fluent than it was at other times. We discussed it directly (Sabat, 2001, p. 304):

SRS: I wonder if, when you're taking a walk, you have fewer problems finding words.

DR. M: Yes, probably. But well you see, I, I'm the teacher, not the, the thing, and uh, uh, being a teacher uh, wasn't, isn't, something very ... it's just I guess what it is, and I have the role of a person who, and maybe I'm losing some of that too.

SRS: So when we were taking a walk you had a different role in the sense that you were leading ...

DR. M: Um hum

SRS: guiding, showing . . .

DR. M: And I, and I've, don't have very much of that now.

She spent decades of her life teaching and guiding young people of college age, so the Self 3 persona of professor/guide/mentor was deeply woven into her being. The problems with her memory and with finding/recalling and pronouncing words that were caused by AD created social circumstances that prevented her from receiving the cooperation she needed to construct a Self 3 other than "Alzheimer's patient." This was something about which she felt great antipathy, for it not only limited her socially but also affected her ability to speak fluently and to be with people in a natural way. As she herself stated, "Sure, I can handle myself. . . . When I try not to let myself be presented as an Alzheimer's, I'm very different" (p. 305). Here, we appreciate (1) her saying clearly that she tries to reject being positioned solely as a "victim of disease" with all the defects that that entails and (2) her awareness of what being put in that position does to her ability to express herself as she would prefer.

I made it a point to recognize and honor her academic achievements, some of the many Self 2 attributes in which she took pride. Rather than positioning her as an "Alzheimer's patient," I was speaking to her as an academic person of great intellectual achievement, and this allowed for the construction of her Self 3 persona of professor and colleague, which opened up the possibility of enlivening conversation that she always enjoyed greatly and missed terribly in her present life. She created the opportunity for me to speak to her support group about the strengths retained by people diagnosed with AD, and in the aftermath, we discussed what happened at that meeting. In that conversation, she encouraged me to use in my research what I had learned in that meeting. I agreed that that would be excellent, and she said with great enthusiasm (p. 306),

DR. M: I knew that! *I knew that, I knew that it gives you just what you're looking for. So uh, and I think it gives, gives the group some.*

SRS: Yes, indeed! I think we learn more about what people *can* do (when we observe them) in very rich social settings.

DR. M: Um hum, *and you can have it for the next uh . . . paper.*

In this exchange, Dr. M was truly being a supportive senior colleague/mentor, as she encouraged me to use what I had learned in writing my "next paper" or, in other words, my next professional journal article. And, in acting this way, she displayed tremendous enthusiasm not only for what I was doing as a researcher but also because she was able to function as the academic, the professor, who loved having this kind of interaction with what would be a "junior colleague," given the difference in our ages. She was living in the moment, excited about the research and all it meant to both of us, for we were conversing as would good colleagues and she was able to live this moment feeling very much "herself."

Constructing a valued Self 3 persona is possible also for someone whose life was quite different from that of Dr. M. Mrs. D, diagnosed as being in the moderate to severe stage of AD, was a high school graduate who was reared in a show business family and knew all the old songs from stage and screen and possessed a great sense of humor. Her brother was a professional stand-up comedian who had performed on television and in nightclubs. She did not put a premium on speaking eloquently or gracefully, often making jokes about her errors of speech when she made them. With the cooperation of the participants and staff at the adult day center she attended 4 or 5 days a week, she constructed the Self 3 persona of "Life of the Party" as she kept other participants as well as the staff laughing heartily and joining her in sing-a-longs that brought great pleasure to everyone. She was also very supportive of others, especially those who were ill and had been away from the day center for some time, for upon their return she would welcome them with great warmth (thus revealing also her memory of them and the fact that they had been gone for some time). The staff saw how wonderful she was with people, and so they worked with her to create another Self 3 persona, "Liaison Between Staff and Participants," to help new attendees become part of the center's community of people. As well, she was very sensitive to the emotional needs of others and worked to bring cheer to those who felt sad. Her Self 2 attribute of wanting to help others found yet another outlet as she, with the cooperation of people at the National Institutes of Health, became a volunteer subject in drug trials even though it meant being faced with her frequent inability to answer questions correctly on the standard tests that were among the outcome measures in the drug efficacy trials. She was very clear about her reasons for doing this work: "I could have said, 'no', but believe me if I can help me and my fe (fellow) man, I would do it" (Sabat, 2001, p. 300).

The effect of the cooperation of others on Mrs. D's ability to construct a valued Self 3 persona at the day center was underscored even more clearly by the lack of cooperation she received at home from her husband, who truly loved her deeply. Unfortunately, he unwittingly saw her primarily as a person diagnosed with AD and focused a great deal more on her dysfunctions than on her strengths, to the degree that he seemed to be unaware of the kind and generous motives behind some of her actions. For example, they slept in different bedrooms, with Mr. D's bedroom closer to the bathroom. At night, when Mrs. D got up to use the bathroom, she always used the one in the basement instead of the bathroom steps away from her bedroom. Mr. D was upset that she failed to flush the toilet in the basement bathroom, as he discovered every morning. When I asked Mrs. D why she did not use the bathroom on the main level of the house, she said, "My husband is a very light sleeper," implying that she did not want to risk awakening him by using the bathroom close to his bedroom. Thus, Mrs. D was limited at home to the Self 3 of "burdensome AD patient" and was generally sullen and quiet there. One could say that she appeared to be two different people: the life of the party, liaison between staff and new participants at the day center and the relatively uncommunicative, sad person at home. Such striking, *consistent* differences could not be the result of the variability in performance that results from brain damage. Rather, they were due to the social influences of other people.

Thus, we see that among the important effects of cooperating with the person diagnosed so as to construct valued and meaningful Self 3 personae are

- decreasing social isolation;
- supporting the ability of the person to give to and receive from others;
- supporting the ability to have varied experiences in day-to-day life;
- allowing the person to feel fulfilled in ways similar to those that he or she sought and achieved in the past;
- helping the person develop new and potentially rewarding personal relationships;
- helping the person to avoid the social misunderstanding that stems from limiting him or her to the social identity of "Alzheimer's patient" or, worse, "demented patient"; and
- providing care partners with the delight of seeing their loved one enjoying good moments, thus replacing the sadness and stress that care partners often feel with the fulfilling delight and calm that they so well deserve.

In addition, we see that many of the diagnosed person's lifelong strengths and history of adaptation and coping styles can remain alive even though the dysfunction in explicit memory, calculation, language, and the like is serious enough to meet the criteria for a diagnosis of dementia. Tapping into the person's remaining abilities can be tremendously helpful in strengthening the process of resilience as well as improving the quality of life of everyone concerned. Unfortunately, it is often the case that the person diagnosed is referred to in the mass media as well as in everyday conversation among people as "an Alzheimer's patient," and this is not helpful at all.

Why is it a disservice to the person diagnosed to be called "an Alzheimer's patient"?

A person is a patient only in relation to a health care professional. The physician–patient or dentist–patient or nurse–patient relationship is a particular kind of social relationship that differs in important ways from other social relationships. Of course, it is perfectly fine for medical professionals to refer to those whom they treat as their patients. What I address here is the tendency for people other than medical professionals to refer to people diagnosed as "Alzheimer's (or dementia) patients." For example, a very intelligent spousal care partner approached me and introduced herself after I had given a lecture. She then introduced her husband by saying, "This is my husband. He's the patient." Clearly, he was far more than just "the patient," but this was the term that she used to introduce him to me.

Although I addressed some aspects of this matter previously, it is worth revisiting it in the context of a person's social self. Let's examine some aspects of what it means to be a patient. Patients are

- recipients of care;
- managed, treated, and told what to do by health professionals and others;
- subservient—in a junior social position to health care professionals who have knowledge and power over them;
- dependent—they cannot make all sorts of decisions without permission; and

- limited-dementia patients are often not viewed as people who have meaning-making abilities, whose actions are driven primarily by the meaning of social situations. Rather, they are seen within a storyline of dysfunction, and much of what they do is often attributed to disease-produced symptoms.

On the other hand, persons are

- givers as well as recipients of care;
- not subservient, can be on an equal social plane with others, and can be junior or senior to others;
- interacted with as opposed to managed;
- able to exercise independence; and
- able to make meaning and act on the basis of the meaning of the situations they encounter.

To refer to someone as an "Alzheimer's patient" creates a label for the person, and this label clearly emphasizes one particular Self 2 attribute of that person (Alzheimer's diagnosis) and one particular Self 3 persona (a "patient"). A person is much more than a patient and has many more attributes than just his or her diagnosis. Indeed, the diagnosis entails only the dysfunctional Self 2 attributes the person has—the areas in which he or she has sustained losses. Clearly, a person has attributes other than his or her losses, such as his or her many positive attributes or strengths. So there is a yawning gap between being a patient and being a person.

It would be rather absurd, for example, to introduce one of your friends to someone by saying, "This is my friend Pat. Pat is a dental patient." It is true, as it turns out, that Pat is a dental patient, but only in relation to his or her dentist, and there is much more to Pat than "patient-hood." To refer to someone as a patient also has the great potential to result in the lack of cooperation that is needed from others for that person to construct a Self 3 (other than "Alzheimer's patient") that is valued by that person and others as well. It will affect how others view the person and can easily result in putting limits on the ways in which others treat that person and thereby limit that person to "patient-hood" and being seen primarily in terms of an attribute that he or she finds cause for sadness, grief, and anguish.

Another reason why referring to someone as an "Alzheimer's patient" is problematic is the increased likelihood that the person will begin thinking of him- or herself primarily as a patient. Recall that Bill, in Lisa Snyder's support group, referred to people with AD as "patients." The problem with this is illustrated vividly in the story of the late actor, Christopher Reeve. In the aftermath of the equestrian accident that left him quadriplegic, Reeve wanted to end his life because he did not want to go on living with that physical condition. His wife prevailed on him to wait some time, see how he feels then, and that if he still wanted to end his life, she would help him. It turned out that in the time that followed, Reeve did extraordinary work to raise public awareness about spinal cord injuries, established the Christopher and Dana Reeve Foundation for research and improving the quality of life for people with injuries such as his and other types as well, lobbied Congress for funding on stem cell research to ameliorate spinal cord injuries, and more. The list of his tireless and inspiring efforts is extraordinary.

The point of this story is simple yet tremendously important. Someone who knew that Reeve wanted to end his life in the aftermath of the accident asked him how he explained the fact that he went on to do such extraordinary work on behalf of others. He said the first step in reclaiming his life was that "I had to stop being a patient and start being a person." In other words, Reeve was saying that when he identified himself as being a patient, he was not mentally capable, mentally free, to consider doing anything on behalf of others. He certainly could not begin to see the possibilities of exercising his will and summoning the energy that would be necessary to do that kind of work. He is telling us that identifying himself as a patient rendered him essentially impotent in the social world but that identifying himself as being a person freed him to engage the world and work for the benefit of others, actually achieving significant goals for others as well as for himself in the process.

How a person views him- or herself, as a patient or as a person, can have a tremendous effect on what the person thinks is possible in life. If a person with dementia views him- or herself as a patient and continues to do so, it will be far more difficult to find some optimism with which to approach life and far less likely for the person to find a path to improving the quality of his or her life. All this means that the process of resilience will be essentially stopped before it can begin.

There is a further complication for the person diagnosed, however, for we must remember that unlike the person with dementia, Reeve's injury did not involve brain damage. His ability to communicate through considered, elegant speech was intact, as were the rest of his cognitive abilities. He was able to use those abilities to reposition himself in the eyes of others who heard him speak and was therefore given the cooperation from others to construct a Self 3 persona (e.g., "Advocate for People with Spinal Cord Injuries") that was valued by him as well as by everyone who heard him speak or heard about the work he was doing. Furthermore, as a result of being able to do that work, he was viewed with great admiration and respect. The situation facing the person diagnosed with dementia is quite different, however.

The person with AD, for example, may have difficulty finding the words he or she wishes to use to express thoughts, may have difficulty pronouncing those words, and may need the patience and facilitative help of others in order to communicate. As a result, it can be far more difficult for this person to succeed in repositioning him- or herself as being a person as long as others continue to view him or her as a patient and fail to provide the facilitative help that is required for communication and mutual understanding to occur.

One important factor that contributes to sustaining the view of the person diagnosed mainly as a patient is the frequent habit of speech that is exemplified by speaking of "the Alzheimer's (or dementia) patient" instead of "the person with Alzheimer's disease." In the former expression, the word "Alzheimer's" is emphasized, and "patient" is clearly connected with medical matters, so this way of speaking about someone focuses only on the type of medical problem he or she has—which is only one of his or her many attributes. In the latter expression, "the person" is emphasized. In order for people with dementia to avoid viewing themselves primarily as "patients," all of us must change the way we speak so as to emphasize "the person" who just happens to have a diagnosis but who clearly possesses many other attributes that are healthy and can contribute positively to the person's sense of self-worth.

This situation is quite similar, in its social and psychological dynamics, to the way we create negative stereotypes about aging. I do not remember hearing the following expression until perhaps the 1990s at the earliest, but it seems that nowadays we refer frequently to errors or faults as "senior moments," thereby reinforcing the negative stereotype. When we speak of and view a person as being the "Alzheimer's patient," we are far more likely to interpret what he or she says and does as a species of dysfunction or some kind of symptom instead of something that could be perfectly appropriate, normal, or healthy. So an "Alzheimer's patient" wanders, whereas he or she, as "a person diagnosed with AD," takes a walk.

At a private group home for people with AD in a Maryland suburb of Washington, DC, there is a secure area outside the house that is part of the property, fenced off from the rest of the neighborhood, where the residents can walk about or sit on benches if they wish. The professional staff refers to this area as "The Wander Garden." Why is it "The Wander Garden" instead of "The Garden"? One answer is that medical professionals operate the house, and they view the residents principally as being "Alzheimer's patients." The residents are therefore assumed to be wandering when they are walking about, for they are seen mainly in terms of the pathological effects of AD. The residents somehow cannot simply go for a walk as would any otherwise healthy person. They "wander." This is but one example of how using the language of pathology can characterize people perpetually. It is as if a person diagnosed with dementia cannot possibly do something that a person deemed healthy does (or even what the same person did before being diagnosed), even though there is no logical or medical reason for that interpretation. People take walks. Even people with AD take walks because, after all, they are people too.

Why can describing walking as "wandering" have a negative effect on resilience?

The interpretation of perfectly normal human actions, walking being just one of them, as being pathological can have profoundly negative effects on resilience for a number of reasons. I used walking here purely as an example that can be applied also to any number of things we do frequently.

First, in order for a person to remain optimistic and engaged with others in relationships that involve mutual giving and receiving (both of which are important factors in resilience), healthy others in the diagnosed person's life must be attentive to and supportive of the person's strengths. Clearly, when healthy others frequently see pathology in the diagnosed person's actions, even when those actions are normal and healthy, they are not being attentive to and supportive of the person's strengths. Indeed, they are ignoring the person's strengths. This hardly supports the diagnosed person's feelings of optimism. Indeed, it could crush those feelings.

Second, those who view the person as a patient only and see only pathology in his or her actions do not cooperate in the creation of relationships that are mutually giving and receiving, which is another important part of the process of resilience. Rather, they cooperate in constructing relationships that involve only their giving to the person diagnosed, whom they see as a "patient." Even with the best of intentions, this results in the person diagnosed feeling increasingly more burdensome and ashamed because he or she is not allowed to reciprocate in kind and thereby show gratitude in the form of doing good deeds in one way or another.

Third, the pathologizing of normal acts can also have a negative effect on the diagnosed person's feelings of self-worth. This can inspire feelings of sadness, even depression, thereby having a negative effect not only on the diagnosed person's quality of life but also on the quality of life of his or her care partners. Indeed, care partners who fail to see and support their loved one's strengths will likely automatically underestimate their loved one's abilities, not involve their loved one in decision-making tasks, and thereby not work to help their loved one maintain as much independence as possible. These care partners are more likely to become angry or resentful about "the bad dream" they are living, especially given that they believe that they have to take charge of everything.

Another example of what can be viewed as a strength, even an instance of creativity, occurred in an interaction that one of my advanced seminar students had with a participant at an adult day center. These students, including Jared Giordano, spent 3 hours each week at the day center interacting with and learning from the participants, many of whom were diagnosed with dementia of the Alzheimer's type. Jared had established an especially warm, caring connection with one of the participants thus diagnosed, an 82-year-old woman. As he was about to leave the center one day, Jared was saying goodbye to people and, as he said goodbye to Mrs. N, she said, "I am happy to love you."

Usually, people say, for example, "I love you" or "I'm happy to know you." It is rare (first time for Jared and first time for me) to hear someone say, "I am happy to love you." It would be rather easy to view this sentence from a pathological standpoint and say that it is an incorrect juxtaposition of two thoughts and, therefore, a reflection of the language-related problems caused by AD. Interestingly, however, Mrs. N really did convey something that is fundamentally true but rarely acknowledged so openly: that we are happy to feel love for another person. In a sense, one could say that she used the language creatively, and that begs us to ask whether people with dementia can be creative and appreciate creativity in other people.

Can people with dementia be creative and appreciate the creativity of others?

The past 15 years have witnessed much increased attention paid to creativity as expressed and as appreciated by people diagnosed with AD and other dementias. John Killick (2016) reported an example of the creative use of language by a woman in her 80s who lived in a dementia care unit. As he walked through the lounge area of the unit, the woman said to him, "If you're not careful, you'll spend your days in the land of the striped sunshine" (p. 179). This sentence is clearly open to interpretation, but my first reaction upon reading this was that the "land of the striped sunshine" was jail—where the windows have bars. When the sun shines through those windows, the bars cast shadows that are parallel lines on the floor or wall, thus "stripes" in appearance. And, of course, you will wind up in jail if you misbehave, if "you're not careful." Alternatively, one can visualize looking toward a window with bars while the sun is shining through and seeing stripes (the bars) surrounded by sunlight, and again there is "striped sunshine." Now, it must be remembered, as Killick frequently reminds us, "that in interpreting the meaning of the language of people with dementia, we need to get away from the literal and look at the symbolic" (Killick, personal communication). This is certainly true of the way people appreciate poetry and prose, so why should it not apply also to what people with dementia say?

Yet another example of appreciating and understanding what people diagnosed say is Elinor Fuchs's (2005) comment about something her mother, diagnosed with AD, said:

Mother exclaimed, "We can do it!" 30 times in 10 minutes on her 84th birthday, radiating a zany good cheer. By this time I was assigning the plays of Gertrude Stein to my students. If Stein could raise repetition to an art form, if Beckett and Philip Glass could do it, why not relax and enjoy it when it came from Mother?

Fuchs makes an excellent point here that I believe should be taken very seriously. That is, we need to ask ourselves the following: If the same thing spoken by the person with AD was, instead, spoken by someone whom we believed not to be diagnosed with AD or another type of dementia, would we see it as an example of pathology and cause for worry? Even further, in line with Fuchs's idea, if we were told that a famous poet uttered those words, would we automatically assume them to reflect some kind of brain damage? Or would we assume that the poet was trying to convey something that we were unable to understand immediately? In these questions, we encounter the very powerful idea that our assumptions about people can affect our interpretation of what they say and do. The famous artist or poet is considered "creative"; the person diagnosed with AD "shows evidence of linguistic pathology." There are clearly gray areas in these often overlapping domains, and we must be open to acknowledging them before immediately pathologizing what someone says or does simply because the person has a particular Self 2 attribute such as a diagnosis of dementia.

Killick has spent a great deal of time conversing with people diagnosed and writing down what they say. Although he does some editorial work on their words, he never adds his own. He has returned them in the form of poetry to the people in question, and in some instances, he has received permission to publish some of the poems (Killick, 1997, 2000, 2008). In a 2016 book chapter he wrote about creativity and people with dementia, Killick reports discussing his work with Ian McQueen, who was 59 years old and in an early stage of dementia at the time of their conversations. McQueen said quite clearly that these conversations were opportunities to "get things off his chest," reminding me of Dr. B thanking me for allowing him to "ventilate" and of the great value of therapeutic conversation with others that people diagnosed often sorely need. More to the present point about creativity, though, Killick refers to an occasion on which McQueen lost the thread of what he was saying and commented, "Look, the little creature, it's running along the skirting-board and disappearing with my thought" (Killick, 2016, p. 192), as if some mouse was absconding with McQueen's thought and running away along the "skirting-board," or baseboard. At the outset of their association, McQueen was skeptical about the idea of making poems out of what he said, but by the end of their collaborative work, McQueen changed his mind about what poetry could do and indicated as much by saying, "A poem is something that feels into my psyche. It is where it comes out and where it ends up—essence of essences. What matters to me is the 'me'-ness of it" (p. 193). McQueen here affirms the powerful meaning he derived from seeing his words become poetry and how they expressed the essence of his thoughts and thereby reflected him: the "me-ness of it." This is yet another example of how it is possible to help people diagnosed to express themselves in a way that is accurate and gives them pleasure. In this incident, we see that our interdependence as people is clear, as is how one can discern meaning and create a satisfying collaborative relationship by listening actively and sensitively to what persons diagnosed say.

Among the many important aspects of Killick's work and that of other researchers who have explored creative expression with people with dementia is that there is no situation in which the person diagnosed can be "wrong" such as they can be on standard tests of cognitive ability or when asked pointedly by care partners to recall recent events. When the situation is such that one cannot be easily embarrassed or feel anxiety, the chances for active engagement and freedom of expression are greatly improved and the possibility of "flow" (Csikszentmihalyi, 1990) is enhanced.

Another example of this is Heather Hill's (2003) use of creative dance with people diagnosed. In four videotaped sessions with Elsie, an 85-year-old woman diagnosed with moderate dementia who had been admitted to a psychiatric hospital for assessment and possible placement in a long-term care home, striking results emerged when Elsie was encouraged to move with music played by a musician. After the sessions, Elsie viewed the videotapes of herself. In addition to the improvement (clearly reflecting the benefit of previous experience and, hence, memory) in the quality and form of her movement, Hill reported that Elsie indicated that she valued dance by saying, "Thank you for bringing me out of my shell"; "It's brought the dullness out from me ... to the brightness"; and "I think it's brought me out. ... Wake up" (p. 39).

Although she was diagnosed as being in the moderate stage of dementia, Elsie was tremendously responsive to the music and able to organize and improve her bodily movements with practice. Furthermore, she reflected on the meaning and significance of the experience. For all her explicit memory dysfunction as measured by diagnostic tests, she was still able to say that the music and dance brought her out of her shell. This obviously showed that she recalled the fact that she had been in something of a shell previously (clearly there was no "memory loss" about that) and not as fully expressive as she knew herself capable of being. As well, she expressed gratitude for the help she received in aiding her to emerge as she did, thereby demonstrating the ability to assign a positive meaning or value to the experience, as would someone who is a semiotic subject—whose actions are driven by the meaning that situations hold. Hill (2003) remarked that the image she had of Elsie was that "of a person in a state of ease with herself rather than of disease and fragmentation" (p. 39). Perhaps, in addition to being in a situation in which she could not be "wrong," the music gave Elsie a "pattern" within which she could fit gracefully and thereby express herself in ways that she could not in the rather sparse, relatively unstimulating environment of the psychiatric hospital where she was residing at the time.

Similar to Hill's work, a group of clowns in the United Kingdom, known as the "Elderflowers," employ humor in working with people diagnosed with dementia to encourage communication in creative ways. Humor opens channels of communication that can spontaneously shift focus so as to include serious topics before returning to something humorous again and so on. One of the tactics used by the group is that its members always fail in doing whatever it is they attempt to do. In addition to provoking laughter, this shows them to be vulnerable, an important attribute that they share with those diagnosed (as well as with all human beings), thereby emphasizing that aspect of the common ground between them. It is important to note that the Elderflowers' function is not simply to provide entertainment. Rather, as Killick (2012) notes, they attempt to use aspects of play to stimulate playfulness in people diagnosed. As a result, there is laughter that then stimulates the formation of genuine, spontaneous, person-to-person connections that are meaningful for everyone. Not only is the interaction meaningful in the moment but also it is memorable, and this is another example of why the term "memory loss" is worthy of being removed from everyday usage. The use and virtue of play to engage people with dementia and provide enlivening moments has been explored well by Killick (2012).

One week after the Elderflowers performed, Killick (2016) visited a hospital to assess their impact and had the following interaction with a woman diagnosed with dementia in the moderate stage:

I showed Vera a photograph of the two actors she had met with in the session a week previously. I reminded her of their names: "Honey Bunch" and "Sweetie Pie." Then I produced a red nose from my pocket similar to the ones they had worn, and to the one she had been lent by them on that occasion. She took it from me and put it on. "I think the noses are good," she said. Then, handing it back, she told me: "Put it away. I wouldn't like it to be harmed. Till they come again." She pointed to the photograph: "They're beautiful children. They must be full of fun. They don't make me feel sad. I'm always very pleased to see them." She went on to point to the male actor: "Someone he loved very much might have died, so he's sad too in a way. They're definitely actors. I talk to them and they talk to me nicely. They play with me, chase me, and I pretend to run very fast. They make me laugh, but only as an act. I like to join in, in very small bits, correcting them. They are my friends, I like them very much." (p. 188)

When people diagnosed are engaged in a lively way that involves a range of emotions, including humor, it turns out to be psychologically valuable for everyone. This is especially true when the performers display their own vulnerability so as to connect with that of the people diagnosed. For people diagnosed, new and pleasant memories are made, and for some, it means emerging from the "shells" in which they often find themselves for lack of experiences with engaged and engaging people. In terms of benefiting from the active, creative engagement of their emotions, people diagnosed with AD and other forms of dementia are no different from the way they were in healthier days.

The importance of the Elderflowers displaying vulnerability by "failing" to do a number of things as part of their performance is worth discussing further. People diagnosed can be especially aware of their present inability to do things that, in years gone by, they always did easily, and they can react with embarrassment, anger, and sadness. By acting out "failure" in a humorous way, the Elderflowers bring some humor to failure and in so doing perhaps make failure a bit less onerous. Perhaps it even encourages people to laugh at themselves in a healthy way. In the process, the performers put themselves in what could be an "empathetic" position and laugh at themselves while they are inspiring laughter in people diagnosed. At the same time, the laughter they inspire is uplifting, genuine, and enjoyed especially by people who have missed laughing in their day-to-day lives. There is yet another side to being vulnerable, though, that friends and care partners can apply to situations in everyday life.

Admitting to one's vulnerability can help create authentic spontaneity with people diagnosed. At times in my conversations with Dr. M, I truly did not fully understand what she was trying to say to me, even when I used indirect repair and other facilitative methods. At those moments, I found that asking her for her help was an especially good thing to do. I would say, "Help me, please," and that was another way to make us equal partners in the situation. I had many opportunities to help her, but she was now aware that she could be of help to me, thereby giving her some social "capital" in the interaction and the feeling that she was an equal contributor. This turned out to be very important to her sense of self-worth, feelings of optimism, and, therefore, her resilience. She also helped me!

There are yet other forms of creativity that have been explored with people diagnosed. A number of researchers have noted that participation in programs wherein creative expression is encouraged provides increased opportunities for social interaction and communication (Allan & Killick, 2000; Basting, 2006; Basting & Killick, 2003), and the positive effects of those increased opportunities are experienced by care partners as well (Fritsch et al., 2009).

One of the more recently developed interventions involving creativity was founded by Elizabeth Lokon at the Scripps

Gerontology Center at Miami University of Ohio and is called Opening Minds through Art (OMA). OMA is an intergenerational art program in which participants are not confronted with failure. The program consists of 60-minute weekly art-making sessions over the course of 12 weeks. Each person diagnosed with dementia is paired with a trained student volunteer who provides assistance and encouragement but who neither completes the artwork nor makes esthetic decisions for the person/artist. Art projects are more along the lines of abstract or nonrepresentational art involving materials such as rice paper, dyes, ink, and bubble wrap and different painting techniques including the use of brushes, pipettes, or paint rollers. Participants in the program have made paintings based on the work of the Russian abstract painter Wassily Kandinsky and the American abstract expressionist artist Jasper Johns. They have also created landscapes by using torn tissue paper and collages depicting the "deep sea" environment through the use of watercolors and netting that is used so as to resemble deep-sea plants and animals. Some participants in the OMA program at the Cedar Village Retirement Community in Mason, Ohio, have glazed ceramic tiles (Lokon & Dana, 2014). The program ends with a public exhibit of the work at a local gallery, thus calling positive attention to the work and strengthening the participants' feelings of accomplishment, self-worth, and appreciation by others.

The OMA program is unlike the traditional structured or recreational activities often provided at day centers and nursing homes that have as their goal the improvement of so-called problematic behavior. It is clearly nothing like having people color something "inside the lines," do childlike "cut-and-paste" activities, or make something they are told to make with some craftlike materials. On the contrary, the OMA program and others of its ilk (Rusted, Sheppard, & Waller, 2006) aim to enhance the participants' quality of life and that of their care partners. Toward that end, the OMA program focuses on the participants' needs for psychologically important facets of life, such as attachment, inclusion, comfort, occupation, and identity. These factors are particularly important with respect to the enhancement of resiliency. Lokon and colleagues report that participants are more engaged in and demonstrate greater pleasure from the program than has been found in other programs that purport to aim at similar goals (Sauer, et al., 2016). One possible reason for this is that the OMA program involves a one-to-one ratio of participant to volunteer, thereby giving the participants focused attention and the possibility of developing a strong bond with another person. Another possible reason is that the volunteers are very mindful about the participants feeling in control of the way the art project develops and gaining confidence to try new things, taking creative risks because one cannot be wrong or fail in this program. For people diagnosed, who have felt an increasing loss of control of many aspects of their lives, this feature is especially important because it encourages independent action and the assertion of the person's desire and will in choosing colors, textures, and designs. Likewise, for people whose social worlds have become increasingly restricted and who have experienced isolation, having a new and developing connection with another interesting and interested person who is respectful and supportive of the diagnosed person's strengths is especially enlivening. Indeed, the feeling is mutual, for the student volunteers report that they experience a truly pleasurable working relationship or friendship with the OMA participants diagnosed with dementia (Lokon, Kinney, & Kunkel, 2012).

The positive effects of the program are apparent to family care partners and professionals alike. For example, a Licensed Practical Nurse at the Westover Retirement Community said, "OMA brings out a different side that we don't usually see during the rest of the day," and an activities specialist at the Berkeley Square community stated, "It lets us see how much they're capable of." The daughter of a 99-year-old Westover resident said, "I'm amazed at what my mother does" (Lokon & Dana, 2014, p. 4). In other words, the daughter in this case did not expect that her mother was capable of doing what she did—and we must ask ourselves: What led to that expectation in the first place? What effect might that expectation have had on how the daughter treated her mother? How many others in the woman's social world shared that expectation, and what were the effects? Clearly, the OMA staff did not have such limited expectations, and their work was more effective as a result.

Can this type of program have a positive effect on the selfhood and resilience of people diagnosed?

One additional element of the OMA program is that the participants diagnosed with dementia are positioned as friends/ mentors of a sort—in that they have the opportunity to impart to others some of the wisdom they have gained in their lives, thereby making the relationship with the student volunteers truly reciprocal, which is another factor involved in resilience. Having the opportunity to be helpful to others, thereby giving life meaning, along with experiencing and expressing autonomy (as in creating the work of art) were of utmost importance to people diagnosed with dementia (Scholzel-Dorenbos et al., 2007), and the OMA program provides both admirably.

Yet another important result emerged from a further study of the OMA program. Yamashita, Kinney, and Lokon (2011) compared the attitudes of students who took a gerontology course and also completed a service-learning component of the course (the OMA project) to those of another group of students who took the same gerontology course without the service-learning component. The students who participated in the OMA component reported far more positive attitudes toward older adults than did the students who did not participate in the service-learning (OMA) component. Indeed, the attitudes of the latter group of students were significantly less positive about working with people diagnosed with dementia. In a sense, then, actually working with people diagnosed with dementia in an authentic relationship that (1) emphasized cooperation, (2) kept the diagnosed person's autonomy foremost in mind, and (3) allowed for mutual learning, conversation, and sharing of thoughts and beliefs all worked to improve young peoples' attitudes toward those diagnosed. It stands to reason that the same type of program would have similar effects if it involved older adults.

This kind of authentic connection entails focusing on the diagnosed person's strengths (positive Self 2 attributes) and the construction of a valued Self 3 persona for the diagnosed person. Both help to dispel the influence of the powerful negative stereotypes as well as the stigma about dementia and thereby can enhance the diagnosed person's resilience.

Is there other evidence that cooperative work can reduce stigma?

Harris and Caporella (2014) found similar results in their study of the value of an intergenerational choir involving students, people diagnosed with AD and mild cognitive impairment, and their care partners. In order to enhance the interaction between all participants, during rehearsals the group was seated in a circle such that everyone could see everyone else. Each student was paired with a person diagnosed and his or her care partner. Before rehearsals began, there was time devoted to socialization, conversation, and stretching exercises to "warm up." This allowed all participants to get to know one another better during the 8-week period of the study and to come to see one another as people first rather than as categories such as "old" or "diagnosed with AD." The music was chosen so as to appeal to everyone and included songs by the Beatles and James Taylor, as well as folk music such as the song "We Shall Overcome." The students' understanding of AD and of people diagnosed was enhanced greatly by the experience of working cooperatively with people diagnosed and their care partners. One student said,

> I have learned that people with AD are really no different from anyone else. ... This experience has changed

the way I perceive people with AD; they can be just as funny and lively as any other person. It has made me put aside the fact that they have AD and treat them equally, as any other elder. (p. 275)

In addition, the students grew more comfortable being with the people diagnosed:

The woman I am paired with reminds me of my grandmother. ... At first I was nervous that she wouldn't remember me on the subsequent weeks of practice, and honestly I'm not sure if she does or not. However, every week she sits next to me and talks with me as if I'm an old friend. And I often forget about the age gap and the disease that divides us, and I look at these people as friends. (p. 276)

Enhanced understanding of the strengths possessed by people diagnosed contributed to the students' ability to look beyond the stigma of the disease and appreciate more deeply the "person the disease has." One student said (Harris & Caporella, 2014),

Although it is sad to admit, I felt my grandma (who has AD) was not "really there" before. Now, I see that even though she has Alzheimer's, she is still my grandma. We need to look beyond the disease and remember the person (who) is still there. (p. 276)

Although before the beginning of the study, only 3 of the 12 students said they would be comfortable spending an afternoon with a family friend diagnosed with AD, by the end of the study, all 12 students said they would be comfortable doing so.

How did people diagnosed and their carers react to being in the intergenerational choir?

For all participants, the experience was positive and greatly reduced the social isolation they experienced (Harris & Caporella, 2014). One participant said, "I love meeting new people, especially young people. They have so much energy. We usually don't have a chance to be with so many young people; we meet old people." Another said, "We all need each other. Listening to everyone's stories and singing together makes me feel less alone" (p. 278). So young and old people, diagnosed and care partners, grew close together while pursuing a common, enjoyable goal, and their enjoyment was so great that they all began coming early to rehearsals and staying later and later at the end. Some of the couples who did not know each other previously began meeting for dinner together. It was clear that a strong and vital community of people was built, and the same feeling of togetherness was powerfully evident in the public concert that was held in front of an audience of 230 people who responded with enthusiastic applause and two standing ovations. There was even a "cast party" afterward; no one wanted to leave at the "official" ending time of 6:00 p.m. and instead stayed an extra hour, and some exchanged e-mail addresses and made plans to meet for dinner in the ensuing weeks.

Although the study by Harris and Caporella (2014) involved only a small number of people, it is still tremendously suggestive of what might be possible for many others. It was clear, for example, that the experience was beneficial to all the participants in very important ways:

1. It decreased the social isolation of the people diagnosed and their care partners.
2. It increased the students' appreciation of the many strengths possessed by the people diagnosed and thereby helped to build warm relationships.

3. The resulting cooperation given by the students made possible the construction of healthy, valued Self 3 personae among those diagnosed. That is, the people diagnosed were no longer seen principally as "Alzheimer's patients."

All of these can, in principle, help strengthen the resilience of those diagnosed as well as that of their care partners. Thus, the engagement of creativity through participation in the intergenerational choir worked to the benefit of all concerned, no matter their age or health status. Indeed, it helped strengthen everyone's humanity and appreciation for one another.

Thus far, we have seen that people diagnosed with AD and other types of dementia can benefit from experiences that engage their creativity and their appreciation of others' creativity in connection with dance, singing, and painting. So this begs the question of whether other arts-based programs are also beneficial.

Are there other arts-based programs that are beneficial to people diagnosed?

Yes, indeed. Kathy Kahn-Dennis (2002) explored the effectiveness of artwork for three people who were diagnosed with dementia, two with the Alzheimer's type, each of whom worked with an art therapist. For each person, the involvement with artwork brought a great deal of satisfaction.

For Mrs. T, aged 82 years at the time, it was a means of revealing a number of her remaining strengths and a reflection of her personality. As she painted a self-portrait, she began to discuss significant narratives about her life. This is certainly meaningful also because as we grow older, we reflect on the meaning of our lives, often via telling stories. Over the course of 2 years, her ability to paint declined, and she commented on that, showing the ability to evaluate her work based on her memory of her ability in years past. As the effects of brain damage became more severe, she began using clay to fashion different shapes and found enjoyment in so doing. She commented, "I really like doing this" and would make gifts of her work to people she held dear.

For Mrs. W, for 8 years, beginning at age 79 years, it was not only a means of portraying her experience of dementia in order to help others understand her point of view but also allowed her to make something without having to rely on verbal skills and involved a social connection with another supportive person, the art therapist.

For Mrs. A, it was a means of tapping her imagination and sense of humor, as well as a means of remaining connected with other people. Even though she did not seem to recall the art therapist or her own paintings from week to week, she found acceptance from others in the art therapy group in the special care center where she resided. She painted more than anyone else at the special care center, and when asked "What do you like about painting?" she replied, "Just doing it. I like to feel it's part of me" (Kahn-Dennis, 2002, p. 258).

Anne Basting (2003) explored the benefits that accrue to people with AD and other forms of dementia when their imaginations are engaged in various ways. One successful program called TimeSlips is an improvisational type of storytelling/creative expression approach that engages people's use of their imagination in groups by creating stories spontaneously as a group (see http://www.timeslips.org). This is yet another approach in which one cannot be "wrong" about what one says and in which care partners and people diagnosed are understood as being equally involved in what transpires. As such, people's strengths are engaged, often including humor, and they experience a sense of accomplishment. These can combine so as to create a feeling of optimism, all of which together can contribute to resilience.

Fritsch and colleagues (2009) investigated the use of TimeSlips with people diagnosed with dementia and living in nursing homes. They found that its use not only increased social interactions among residents diagnosed but also had a very positive effect on the staff's views of people diagnosed. The staff members who participated in the program were less likely to devalue the residents, engaged them more in social interactions, and made more eye contact with them than they did before participation in TimeSlips. When staff members participated with residents in a creative endeavor, they experienced the residents' strengths in ways that they did not before, thereby allowing them to appreciate the residents more deeply and engage them more actively, and this enhanced the quality of life for the residents as well as their carers.

There is much to be gained when people diagnosed with AD or other types of dementia are engaged in ways that tap into their creativity, thereby reducing instances of embarrassment and humiliation while simultaneously allowing their strengths to be revealed and appreciated in enlivening interaction. The resilience of everyone involved can be enhanced, and the selfhood of those diagnosed can be strengthened. All of these positive outcomes are especially important when people diagnosed are living in long-term care homes, which is one of the subjects of Chapter 6.

6

TYPES OF CARE AND
THE ROLE OF SPIRITUALITY

The powerful stigma and negative stereotypes regarding Alzheimer's disease (AD) and other dementias can lead to unnecessary fear, embarrassment, anger, and depression in people diagnosed and their loved ones. The importance of providing education and supportive care that is not influenced by stigma and stereotype cannot be overstated. Even if a drug could halt the progress of AD in those diagnosed and prevent its occurrence in everyone else, there would still be tens of millions of people worldwide with irreversible brain injury due to AD and other diseases that cause dementia and even more people who serve as their familial and professional care partners. Providing enlightened supportive care is therefore of utmost importance, but how care is provided is intimately connected to how people in need are viewed.

Those diagnosed may be viewed primarily as people who have lived many decades of life and who, despite problems due to illness, have dispositions, ways of being, beliefs, and desires that are woven into them so deeply that they cannot be erased entirely by the brain damage that causes AD or other types of dementia. As well, we may view them as people who persist in trying to communicate however they can and who deserve to retain the rights and privileges they always enjoyed as adults until they are shown clearly to be incapable of doing what is required to retain particular privileges, such as driving.

Conversely, they may be viewed as patients, defined primarily by their diagnoses, whose actions are increasingly dysfunctional, who are mostly dominated by pathological symptoms of disease, who are increasingly confused and irrational, and who require medication in order to "manage" their symptoms. Indeed, as the titles of the following books suggest, people with AD are viewed precisely in this manner: *Death in Slow Motion: A Memoir of a Daughter, Her Mother, and the Beast Called Alzheimer's* (Cooney, 2004) and *A Curious Kind of Widow: Loving a Man with Advanced Alzheimer's* (Davidson, 2006). In such cases, persons diagnosed are viewed as compromised so much as to render them unworthy of retaining the rights and privileges they heretofore enjoyed, including the right to be treated with common courtesy and the privilege of being consulted regarding any number of decisions being made within the family, some of which involve them.

It is unfortunate that the latter of the previously mentioned views is still dominant to one or another degree even among some people who try their best to help those diagnosed. We are, however, making progress toward a far more holistic understanding of people with AD and other dementias by telling their stories: examining the people they are and have been and appreciating them and their present state in light of the lives they have lived.

What is a holistic understanding?

A telling example is the case of Frederick C. Hayes, as described by Rebecca Mead (2013). Hayes was a Korean War veteran and a retired trial lawyer who, in his early 80s, was diagnosed with AD and admitted to a long-term care home. He was known by an old friend to have had a strong, argumentative personality for most of his adult life, and professional aides now described him as "combative." He had been moved from one institution to another, none seeming capable of dealing effectively with his aggressive behavior. Not even doses of Haldol, a very strong antipsychotic drug, helped. Living in an "advanced dementia unit," he seemed to be experiencing a great deal of discomfort, but when physicians asked him to rate his level of pain on a scale of 1 to 10, he said that he was not in pain. Still, he fought with nurses' aides, even kicking some. This behavior is often understood, from a medical standpoint, as symptomatic of AD and characterized as "irrational hostility" or "combativeness," which are among the Behavioral and Psychological Symptoms of Dementia (BPSD), as they are called by medical personnel, that result from the brain damage caused by AD. As Mead reported, however, there was much more to Mr. Hayes's actions than that simple interpretation.

How Mr. Hayes acted and what he said seemed to be connected to how other people approached and treated him. For example, when Ms. Tena Alonzo, Director of Education and Research at the Beatitudes Campus, a retirement community in Phoenix, Arizona, encountered Mr. Hayes, something rather different transpired between the two. Ms. Alonzo views people diagnosed with dementia not as "dementia patients" but, rather, as "people who have difficulty in thinking" and whose actions, even if not initially viewed as such, are forms of communication nonetheless. In this sense, her thinking is similar to that of Pia Kontos (whose work was discussed in Chapter 4), who calls our attention to the important ways people express themselves through bodily actions, and it is also reflective of what is called "taking the intentional stance" (see Chapter 4). So, given this way of thinking about people diagnosed, Ms. Alonzo noticed the grimace on Mr. Hayes's face and how he moaned and writhed as he lay in his bed. Assuming that he might be in pain, and that he was able to understand her, she approached him with a non-anxious presence and told him in a soft tone of voice that she was there to help. She then asked if he hurt anywhere, and she moved her hand gently from one part of his body to another. As she did this, she asked, "Do you hurt here?" for each place she touched. When she touched his stomach, he stopped moaning and said, "I hurt so bad."

When Mr. Hayes was given a higher dose of pain medication, he became increasingly more verbal and stopped acting in an aggressive manner.

When we think about Mr. Hayes's previous actions with this in mind, we can begin to understand what may have been happening. Because of the brain damage due to AD, he was unable to tell others that he had terrible pain in his stomach. Why was he unable to tell physicians how he rated his pain on a scale of 1 to 10? Perhaps he was in too much pain to begin thinking about using numbers on a scale to describe the intensity of his pain, or even to understand the point of the question. Perhaps he did not want to deal with people whose questions were only adding to his discomfort. When he was moved in one way or another in order to change his clothing, or if an aide touched him in the wrong place, the pain increased. Unable to use words to indicate that what they were doing was causing him more pain, all he could do to try to stop the actions that were causing him pain was to swat or kick at the people who were moving him around. Simultaneously, the aides who were unwittingly causing him pain did not understand all that. Having been taught from a biomedical-oriented point of view that AD can produce "irrational hostility" and "combative behavior," they assumed that his actions were those pathological symptoms rather than anything caused by what they were doing. That is, they were assuming that his aggressiveness was an instance of BPSD.

This situation illustrates something that Ms. Alonzo said—something that a host of researchers and practitioners have been saying as well and continue to say: "All behavior is communication" (see the discussion on "taking the intentional stance" in Chapter 4) so that for this group of researchers and practitioners, BPSD has come to mean something rather different from the medical meaning. Instead, we see it as Behavioral and Psychological Signs of Distress to acknowledge that people with dementia are often in distress and may express that distress in ways other than via words. Mr. Hayes was experiencing great distress due to the pain he felt and could not control. When people with dementia have difficulty in finding words to use, they rely increasingly on other means. Therefore, how a person behaves can be an expression of pain and discomfort, aversive environmental conditions, or the need for social contact or other stimulation, all of which can be informative if viewed as communicative efforts rather than pathological symptoms. In recent years, many have advocated for an approach that applies this idea to care settings (Allan & Killick, 2014; Brooker, 2012; Brooker et al., 2013; Cohen-Mansfield, 2014; Downs & Bowers, 2014; Elvish et al., 2014; Hughes, 2011, 2014; Hughes & Baldwin, 2006; Hughes, Louw, & Sabat, 2006; Keady et al., 2012; Kitwood, 1995, 1998; Power, 2010; Sabat, 2001). This leads us to a series of questions that are discussed in the following sections.

What types of care are available?

There are different kinds of care for people diagnosed depending on their needs and abilities. For people still living in their own home or in that of a relative, there are programs such as those mentioned in Chapter 5 as well as support groups that meet weekly or biweekly and adult day centers where people with dementia can attend for the day usually on two or more weekdays each week. Adult day centers provide social interaction and programs or activities that are stimulating and can ease the social isolation that many people experience after having been diagnosed. They also give care partners the ability to work, if necessary, or to take care of household business or just have some free time to enjoy on their own without having to worry about the safety and well-being of their loved one (Zarit et al., 2014). For family and spousal care partners, there are also support groups, many of which can be found by contacting the local chapter of the Alzheimer's Association in the United States or the Alzheimer's Society in other countries.

What transpires in support groups for people diagnosed and those for their care partners is very important, as we saw for Bill and his wife in Chapter 5, because each person can experience and react differently to the effects of the disease that causes dementia as well as to the way others treat him or her. People diagnosed and their care partners can learn a great deal by participating in support groups, but ultimately, it is important for each couple, each family, to understand what dementia means for them—in terms of dysfunctions but also, very importantly, in terms of the strengths that remain intact. This is why one needs to understand two other types of care: person-centered and relationship-centered care.

What is person-centered care?

Person-centered care (Brooker, 2006; Cheston & Bender, 1999; Kitwood, 1998) is essentially the opposite of a "one-size-fits-all" approach to care for people diagnosed and can be provided by family members at home or by staff in assisted-living settings and long-term care homes. It focuses first on the person's strengths. Furthermore, it attempts to maximize independence by empowering families so that they are clearly aware of the strengths possessed by the person diagnosed and then interact with their loved one in ways that take advantage of those strengths. This approach is therefore geared toward helping the person diagnosed feel enabled, valued, and socially confident (Younger & Martin, 2000). That is, supporting the person's feelings of self-worth, his or her self-esteem, is understood to be of paramount importance, especially given the terrible stigma that surrounds being diagnosed—the stigma of which the person diagnosed has likely been aware for many years preceding the diagnosis.

The foundation of person-centered care is that one's spouse or parent or sibling or friend who is diagnosed with AD or another type of dementia ought to be loved, respected, and supported for reasons that go far beyond his or her ability to recall what was served for dinner that evening or the name of a particular relative or the ability to use eating utensils properly. Indeed, one should not view a person's ability to recall such things as some "litmus test" of the person's value or knowledge or ability to feel hurt or embarrassed or humiliated. In addition, the way AD or another type of dementia affects a person goes beyond the particular dysfunctions that led to the diagnosis. There is also the person's reaction to the dysfunctions and to the way others act, the personality of the person diagnosed, and his or her life experience and networks of relationships. All of these are taken into account in person-centered care, and some examples can be illuminating.

How does person-centered care look in everyday life?

Some spousal care partners may feel the need to take over various tasks that both people previously divided between them. A person-centered care approach suggests that it is far more beneficial to both people for the person diagnosed to be included in any number of decisions, especially about everyday matters that were always part of their lives together. This is especially true for people in the mild and moderate stages and even some in the severe stage of dementia, depending on the matter at hand. Some people diagnosed will indicate directly that they feel left out of things. For example, one couple had business to conduct in a computer store and, before entering the store, the husband (who was diagnosed with AD) told his wife that he wanted to be the one to tell the service person what was amiss with their computer. He was feeling unhappy about having been left out of a good many decisions and intrafamily situations because his wife had taken over doing a great many things herself, and he did not want to continue feeling that way. Clearly, he made a memory of her having done that and was able to retrieve that memory and apply it to the occasion in question here, thereby showing that he had no memory dysfunction regarding this situation. Thus, for him, taking charge of this situation was important to his sense of self-worth even though his wife had to remind him of what he should say just before they encountered the service person. He needed to show himself and his wife that he was still able to do something that in the past he would have taken care of easily. In addition, he needed to present himself to the service person in a positive way. He was acting out of proper pride and working to maintain self-respect. This person verbalized clearly what he needed from his wife, but not every person diagnosed will address his or her needs that clearly, openly, and calmly. Another person might resent the spouse or adult child for taking over decision-making and other activities but not say anything until after a great many such situations have occurred and then explode with a burst of anger. This way of reacting would likely be consistent with the way he or she reacted in the past, thus exemplifying the idea that a person's dispositions can remain intact long beyond the time of the diagnosis. Naturally, there are exceptions to this idea, such as the person whose brain damage involves parts of the frontal lobes that are involved in the ability to "edit" or inhibit what one thinks. In such cases, a person may utter obscenities even though he or she was a model of decorum in the past.

Another example of person-centered care in everyday life involves Dr. and Mrs. B (see Chapter 3). Dr. B always wrote the checks to pay the household bills. There came a point at which he, diagnosed with AD years earlier, could no longer manage the checkbook. Rather than take over the entire process, Mrs. B continued to ask her husband to sign the checks that she had written. She continued to explain to him which bill was being paid by each check that he signed. In this way, he was still involved in doing something that was always "his" and did not feel excluded or pushed aside entirely in connection with "family business."

These kinds of interactions reflect one of the pillars of person-centered care, *collaboration,* and they also include another pillar, *validation,* which is acknowledging and responding to another person's feelings and emotions. In this way, we see how a partnership between people is maintained, thereby contributing to the emotional well-being of both. When this kind of interpersonal relationship is not allowed to flourish, there can be disadvantages for both people. For example, Mrs. K was diagnosed with AD and Mr. K, her spouse, increasingly took over most of the tasks that his wife formerly carried out (Sabat, 2001). He explained that he did this because he feared that she would fail to do what he asked her to do, and he wanted to "protect" her from the experience of failure (and, presumably, protect himself from the experience of having to watch her fail). Thus, he was doing all this for what we can appreciate as being a good, loving, reason. What he took over doing included setting the table before meals, cooking meals, choosing the clothes she would wear, and even applying her make-up for her in the morning before they went out. It was clear from her actions at the adult day center she attended that she was able to set tables because she did so to help the staff before the lunch meal was served. Mr. K commented that she "smuggled" (his word) make-up with her to the day center. He knew this because she applied it to her face while she was at the center, thereby covering up blemishes that his application of the make-up failed to conceal to her satisfaction. He reported further that her job of applying the make-up was much better than was his, which stood to reason considering that he did not have a great deal of practice doing so and her motor skills remained excellent. I commented to him that it might be a good idea to allow his wife to do all the things that she is still able to do because that would relieve him of some of the work he was taking on himself unnecessarily, thereby adding to his feelings of stress and exhaustion. He readily agreed. Of course, his motivation in doing all he did was of the highest. He was trying to be as supportive of his wife as possible, not realizing that allowing her to do all she was still able to do would be the best way of supporting her. After all, for many decades, his wife always applied her own make-up and always picked out the clothes she would wear before going out of the house (she was always beautifully, tastefully, dressed), and so allowing her to continue to do so would be recognizing her as the able adult woman she was, in fact, still. As well, it would allow her to feel self-sufficient in very important ways and thereby add to her sense of self-worth while simultaneously removing one reason for her to feel depressed and burdensome.

Still other aspects of this cooperative approach are valuable to both care partners. One is related to the sense of *agency* that is involved in the previous examples. Agency refers to a person's feelings of control over actions and their consequences (Moore, 2016), and it involves the benefits of making choices and having clear responsibilities to discharge. Keeping the sense of agency alive in people as they age has been shown to have positive physical and mental effects as well as positive effects on quality of life as a whole in people living in nursing homes (Langer & Rodin, 1976). Conversely, Langer and Rodin found that the reduction of the sense of agency was associated with poor health and negative effects on quality of life. Thus, it stands to reason that when people diagnosed with dementia are given the opportunity to be involved in cooperative work with their care partners, to make choices about things, and to have responsibilities of their own, their experience of a sense of agency will have positive effects in a variety of ways. Connected to agency is the sense of having purpose in life such as participating in aspects of family affairs, including assuming some responsibility for tasks of daily life—for example, signing checks to pay bills (Dr. B) and setting the table, applying one's own make-up, and choosing one's own clothes to wear (Mrs. K).

Interestingly, in a study by Boyle et al. (2012), purpose in life was an important factor in helping to maintain better cognitive function even at more severe levels of AD in terms of brain pathology, as measured on autopsy. These investigators found that among people who had higher levels of purpose in life, even though the brain damage due to the progression of AD had become increasingly more severe over time (more amyloid plaques and greater density of tau tangles per square millimeter in various areas of the brain), there was no concomitant decrease in cognitive ability as measured by a battery of 21 standard tests given annually. That is, whatever is involved in having purpose in life, such as engaging one's sense of agency in a way that contributes positively to one's sense of self-worth because one is doing good for others as well as for oneself, also has positive effects on brain function. In other words, although there was more brain damage in such people, they were able to do more with the brain tissue that remained healthy than would have been possible if they did not have the high level of purpose in life that they did, in fact, have. There may be many reasons for this, including the notion that when we engage life in complex ways (having purpose is a very complex psychological matter, as is learning and being of help to others), there may be an effect on brain tissue such that neurons create increasingly more connections (synapses) among themselves, which can create synaptic or cognitive reserve (Stern, 2012). The increase in the number and complexity of synapses among neurons in the brain allows for more complex functions to be performed than would be possible without synaptic complexity. Thus, creating more complex synapses by using the brain to engage life in complex ways creates what may be seen as a sort of protection such that the brain can withstand more damage without the dire effects than would otherwise ensue.

Therefore, person-centered care can have powerful effects (1) on the diagnosed person's feelings of self-worth, competency, and sense of living up to his or her long-established sense of responsibility to self and others; and (2) on brain function such that increased brain damage has a smaller effect on the person's ability to think in a variety of ways, as measured by standard tests. Person-centered care has been found to have still other positive outcomes.

For example, Richards et al. (2001) learned that when, in a nursing home, a person-centered approach was applied to activities in connection with people's past interests and current abilities, there was an improvement in people's sleep patterns; they spent increasingly less time napping during the day and had more solid sleep at night. That is, when people were engaged in doing things that they enjoyed, rather than in things they considered "mindless" or "beneath them" or just plain "boring," they were involved more deeply, expended more energy, stayed awake longer (because they were engaged in thinking about or doing things they found compelling), napped less, and slept better at night. These results should hardly be surprising. Most of us become sleepy when we are bored or unengaged.

In addition, a person-centered orientation to deal with what was called "agitation" and disturbed sleep patterns among people with dementia had positive effects. When people living in a nursing home were given the freedom to choose when to take their meals, when to go to sleep, the activities in which they would participate, and when to use the toilet, there were decreases in verbal agitation levels, and staff felt less rushed and were better able to interact well with the residents (Matthews et al., 1996). The following must be remembered in connection with this research: (1) The freedom to make choices about these matters is similar to how people have lived most of their lives; (2) exercising choice is an example of agency, and we have noted the benefits of experiencing and exercising agency; (3) when people in nursing homes are not allowed to make the previously mentioned choices, it goes against the way they have lived most of their lives, removes agency, and encourages passivity; and (4) it is therefore hardly surprising that when forced into an extremely regimented way of life that removes the ability to make decisions as in (2), people become increasingly agitated verbally. Who wants to live in a place where one is told it is time to eat, especially if one is not particularly hungry? Who wants to be told it is time to go to sleep, especially if one is not particularly tired? Who wants to be told he or she must participate in an activity in which he or she has little or no interest? In his book *Being Mortal,* Atul Gawande (2014) encapsulated very well the problems inherent in many of the places that purport to provide long-term care: "Our elderly are left with a controlled and supervised institutional existence, a medically designed answer to unfixable problems, a life designed to be safe but empty of anything they care about" (pp. 108–109).

On the level of the self-esteem felt by people diagnosed with dementia, when other people attend to their particular positive attributes/strengths and when they are given the opportunity to express those strengths publicly, they are more likely to maintain feelings of self-worth and simultaneously minimize anxiety, grief, anger, and feelings of being burdensome to their loved ones and professional care partners (Sabat et al., 1999). This, too, should not be at all surprising.

Person-centered care can be provided when people diagnosed are living at home or with loved ones as long as the family care partners are (1) cognizant of the diagnosed person's strengths and (2) do not overlook them or take over all the responsibilities of day-to-day living, including those that the diagnosed person can perform. This does raise an important question, however.

Can person-centered care be provided in a nursing home or long-term care setting?

Clearly, based on some of the research cited previously, it is possible for person-centered care to be provided in a nursing home or long-term care setting, but the fact remains that person-centered care in the United States is not the rule for some important reasons. Specifically, a study extending for a period of more than a year indicated clearly that there are some very serious difficulties involved with the creation of true person-centered care, even in very expensive long-term care settings (Doyle & Rubinstein, 2013). Although many long-term care residential homes market themselves as providing this kind of care, there can be rather striking deviations in what person-centered care actually means and how it is put into effect within a particular care home. When Doyle and Rubinstein interviewed administrators, senior staff, and front-line aides and observed daily life as it unfolded in an expensive long-term care home for people with dementia, they found great variation in the different staff members' understanding of this kind of care. This was likely due to problems in how person-centered care was defined and then communicated within the nursing home hierarchy: Administrators and different staff members had very different ideas about what was involved, and some supervisors appeared, based on how they spoke about the subject, not to be clear at all about its meaning. The few aides who were "people-oriented" themselves, to their credit, delivered person-centered care even if they were not aware of this term or that this was their approach.

For families, this means that it is extremely important to become educated about this kind of care and then to investigate different care homes thoroughly so as to assess whether or not such care is actually provided. There can be a huge gap between what is presented in marketing efforts and the reality of daily life. One must inquire about the home's specific policies regarding matters including personalizing daily routines, such as taking meals, going to sleep, and awakening in the morning; choices provided to residents regarding participation in activities; choices provided among different activities; and the like. It is worth observing if the staff members refer to people living in the home as "patients" or as "residents" because this indicates how people are viewed and, therefore, treated. A few follow-up visits to observe how person-centered care is implemented are also important. This kind of investigation clearly takes time, so many elder care advocates recommend that families do this sort of research long before needing such services for loved ones.

Daunting as this may sound, there is evidence that it is quite possible to provide admirable person-centered care in a long-term care setting. One such setting is the aforementioned Beatitudes Campus in Phoenix, Arizona, which is a multi-level residential home where the residents include people of varying levels of ability who are there for different purposes ranging from rehabilitation to long-term residence. The staff at Beatitudes has incorporated a number of the previously discussed person-centered care features into the residents' daily lives. For example, there is no fixed bedtime or waking up time, and residents can choose when to eat even though breakfast, lunch, and dinner are served at typical times. If someone wants a meal late at night or in the wee hours of the morning, it can be arranged. Beatitudes appears to be run more like a hotel than what is often referred to these days, rather oddly, as a "facility" (Who would yearn to live in a "facility"?) Different hallways are painted different soft, pleasing, calming colors that help residents find their rooms far more easily than if all the hallways were painted the same color. Exits are marked with "Stop" signs rather than garish lights to prevent residents from using those particular doors. There is nothing that even remotely resembles a "one-size-fits-all" approach to care at Beatitudes. The "one-size-fits-all" system so commonly found in long-term care "facilities" is more for the benefit of the often overworked staff than for that of the residents. At Beatitudes, Hershey's kisses and lollipops are often employed when residents appear to be upset or distressed, and these seem far more effective in a variety of ways than using antipsychotic drugs such as Seroquel, whose financial costs are quite significant. Seroquel is essentially a chemical restraint in this context and is not approved, as noted on the company's website, for people with dementia. Just the same, it is still used in nursing homes as a way of controlling the residents and keeping them "quiescent" (or, more accurately, sleepy most of the time) for the benefit of the staff.

Some people with dementia who live in long-term care homes spend a great deal of time walking about, and it is quite common for them to be described as "wanderers," as if "wandering" were a symptom of dementia. When one views taking walks in the context of a person's life, however, a very different picture may emerge. Mead (2013) reported that when she visited the Beatitudes campus, she heard the staff members discussing a rather elegant 80-something-year-old woman who spent most of her days walking for hours in the corridors of the dementia unit. After many hours of walking, it appeared from the way she began to walk so gingerly that her feet hurt. Rather than being a symptom of dementia, her continuous walking was a reflection of the fact that in her long professional life, she worked in retail sales, and therefore spent a great deal of time on her feet, walking throughout the store in which she worked. The fact that she was diagnosed with dementia did not erase her desire to remain active by walking. Doing so was clearly purposeful, healthy for her, and not something even remotely describable as "aimless wandering."

Another example of person-centered care reported by Mead (2013) involved a long-term care resident at the Cobble Hill Health Center in Brooklyn, New York. The man was "a former longshoreman who became enraged at mealtimes; after staff learned that, as head of his family, he had always been served first, they began giving him his meals before the other residents, and the outbursts stopped" (p. 101). This is an excellent example of incorporating aspects of an individual's life story into the system of care provided. Without knowing the man's history, it would have been easy to interpret his outbursts as instances of "irrational hostility" due to dementia and look to pharmacological intervention as a method of calming him down. It is therefore important for everyone to understand the point of view of the people whom they are there to help, for whom they are providing care. Of course, one could rightly say that the man should have known that the home was not the home of his past, that the other residents were not his family, and that the old "rule" of him being served first no longer applied in this setting. Furthermore, one could correctly say that he did not understand this because of the brain damage that resulted in dementia. Both these statements are likely true, but what do we do now? How do we deal with him? Give him tranquilizing drugs? Isolate him from others? It seems best from the standpoint of efficiency and cost (financial and emotional), as well as his social life, to understand his past, serve him first, and thereby eliminate his outrage.

In order to understand the point of view of residents in long-term care, Mead (2013) reported that Ms. Alonzo, the Director of Education and Research, encouraged the staff to experience what residents at typical nursing homes experience. Thus, they spoon-fed food into one another's mouths, had to brush each other's teeth, and the like so as to develop empathy for residents who experience that type of treatment daily. Staff went so far as to wear adult diapers, as do most residents in nursing homes, and thereby experienced the great discomfort of having to sit in wet diapers, as do many nursing home residents, as they wait for staff to help them. As a result, the staff decided not to have most of the residents wear the diapers and began taking residents to the restroom soon after mealtimes instead. Everyone involved was much happier, and the residents were far less agitated thereafter. These exercises helped staff members understand the experience of people with dementia living in long-term care, and it is especially admirable that their reactions were not to impose on others what they themselves found to be objectionable. It is important to note that the staff *did not* assume that their clients with dementia had lost the ability to react to these situations just as they would have during their earlier adult lives.

Still other examples of person-centered long-term care were the subject of an article by Alana Semuels (2015) that focused on the challenges and benefits of building better nursing homes that are made to be more like homes than hospitals, more human and humane than sterile, and more geared toward the comfort and happiness of the residents without sacrificing the staff's ability to provide first-rate care. Indeed, the less sterile the residential home becomes, the lower is the frequency of

Behavioral and Psychological Signs of Distress (BPSD) among the residents and that, in turn, helps the staff greatly.

Another example of the value of a nonsterile environment is found in the work of Edwards, McDonnell, and Merl (2013), who examined the effect of a "therapeutic garden" and an atrium/sunroom on the quality of life of people living in a group home in Australia. There were 10 residents, 7 of whom were diagnosed with AD, 2 with a dementia of unspecified type, and 1 with a mixed dementia. Of the 10 residents, 4 were diagnosed with severe dementia, whereas 3 were diagnosed as being moderate and 3 in the mild stage. Staff and family members indicated that the ability of the residents to enjoy walking outside in a lovely garden and having a welcoming room (sunroom/atrium) to enjoy away from a television improved their quality of life dramatically. Before the atrium/sunroom was constructed, the residents spent a great deal of time in the living room, where the television was located. After the atrium/sunroom was constructed, the residents gravitated there instead. Quantitative measures showed that depression scores declined by more than 10 percent and agitation scores decreased by almost half. These, along with the qualitative measures from interviews, showed that a warm, welcoming environment that allowed for walking and enjoying nature had great value for people with dementia at various degrees of severity.

Person-centered care and a humane living environment are of great value to people living with dementia. Just the same, we live our lives among others, and people diagnosed with AD and other forms of dementia have close relationships with family members. When a person is diagnosed, the effects are not limited to the person in question. They affect the entire family in one way or another. How other members of the family think about and interact with the person diagnosed is very important, just as is how professionals think about and interact with those diagnosed. As a result, it is important to ask what is relationship-centered care.

What is relationship-centered care?

There are many ways to understand the meaning of relationship-centered care. Nolan et al. (2004) introduced a compelling approach, and Adams (2003) and Adams and Gardiner (2005) provided some specific applications. The former group focused their attention on the ways in which caring can be the focus of interpersonal relations, whereas the latter work by Adams and Gardiner involved the way people with dementia are treated in triads—when there are three people involved in a meeting or discussion, one of whom has been diagnosed—as well as among other people.

The basis of relationship-centered care is that "the senses framework" be applied to everyone involved in care-focused relationships: the person diagnosed, family care partners, professional aides, and volunteers. Each of these individuals ought to experience relationships that promote the following: a sense of security (to feel safe), a sense of continuity (people have unique biographies that can be used to provide present and future care), a sense of belonging (having mutually reciprocal relationships and feeling that one is part of a community), a sense of purpose (opportunities to engage in meaningful activities, to pursue meaningful goals, and to exercise choice), a sense of achievement (to feel satisfied with one's efforts and to make a contribution), and a sense of significance (to feel recognized and valued as a person of worth and that one's actions and existence are of importance).

With this framework in mind, Adams (2003) and Adams and Gardiner (2005) suggested a variety of ways to enhance communication in groups of three people so that the person diagnosed has the opportunity to be heard fully while feeling safe and part of a small group conversation rather than feeling apart from or ignored by the others. Examples of conversation-enhancing actions are being sensitive to nonverbal cues, promoting equal participation of the person diagnosed, providing the person diagnosed with opportunities to talk, promoting joint decision-making, and removing distracting stimuli from the venue in which the conversation is taking place.

Along these lines, in Germany, Svenja Sachweh (2008) has worked with people in multilingual environments and has provided some important suggestions for enhancing communication with people with dementia. For example, because the brain damage that produces dementia often robs people of their command of foreign languages, and also of formal, standard versions of their mother tongue learned later in life, it is often preferable to address them not only in their mother tongues but also in the slang, dialect, or informal language they learned in early childhood. Another suggestion that would reflect a person-centered as well as a relationship-centered approach concerns people in the more severe stages of dementia. Sachweh observed that many people with dementia in the late stages can take the words of others literally and may become confused or even agitated by metaphorical or hyperbolic expressions such as "We are going to have a shower now" or "It's raining cats and dogs." She notes as well how word-finding problems can be expressed: A person might replace the target word either with words that have a similar meaning (e.g., saying "fork" instead of "spoon") or with words that sound similar to the target word (e.g., saying "moon" instead of "spoon"). Knowing this can empower care partners by helping them understand what the person diagnosed is trying to communicate and, thereby, allow the conversation to move along smoothly without interruption. Knowing that communication is not limited to the use of words, Sachweh suggests that care partners can find it useful to employ pantomime and gesture to be more easily understood, and if one exaggerates these, one might give everyone something to laugh about. The use of gesture and pantomime and other nonverbal behavior was found to be helpful as well by Sabat and Cagigas (1997) and Hubbard et al. (2002).

When we examine person-centered care and relationship-centered care, it seems that when the former is done well, as it is at the Beatitudes campus, the latter also comes into play as a matter of course. For example, when the staff understood that the reason for the longshoreman's outbursts at mealtimes was not at all irrational given his history, they served him first (person-centered care) and thereby contributed to his feeling of being safe, recognized his unique biography, his being part of a community, and gave him a sense of being valued. Simultaneously, the staff experienced satisfaction with their own efforts, felt that they contributed to his well-being, found a sense of purpose in their actions, and believed that their actions were valuable. Broadly then, when we attempt to provide others with the elements of the "senses framework," we provide them for ourselves as well. It is often true that what empowers a person with AD or another type of dementia has the effect of empowering the care partner, whether that person is a spouse, a sibling, an adult child, or a professional. This quite naturally begs the question, What about the caring for healthy care partners?

What about caring for the healthy care partner?

Healthy care partners also require care. If the person diagnosed lives with a relative, it is clear that the relative in question can easily experience chronic psychological and physical stress for many reasons. Those involved have had long-standing relationships with one another, and the introduction of illness, no matter what it may be, can serve to exacerbate old interpersonal tensions and difficulties in addition to reactions to the current illness and its effects. When the illness causes dementia in a family member, the levels of stress and anxiety can be especially daunting. Thus, it is not uncommon for the healthy care partner to experience burnout if he or she is not (1) well educated about AD or other types of dementia; (2) able to recognize and put to use the cognitive strengths and remaining social abilities of the person diagnosed and include that person in matters that can involve his or her collaboration; (3) taking time away from being "on call" constantly in order to be with a solid network of friends, especially in the case of male care partners, who often have far less experience than women in providing supportive care for others; and (4) organizing a "team" of people to provide help with sundry chores such as mowing the lawn. Having a social life is of tremendous value to otherwise healthy care partners. That social life must extend beyond attending support group meetings, even though these are of great value in many ways, not the least of which is the knowledge that one is not alone. Just the same, having an ongoing social life and valued relationships with friends is extremely important when one is providing support for a loved one. To underscore the need for time "off," researchers have learned that chronic stress can occur from unremitting caregiving wherein the spouse (especially) or adult child or sibling essentially takes over doing almost everything for their relative who is diagnosed with dementia. The ensuing stress can have profoundly negative effects on the immune system, making the care partner increasingly vulnerable to illness, and these effects can last more or less for 3 years after caregiving ceases (Kiecolt-Glaser et al., 2003). Thus, because reducing stress can have powerfully beneficial effects psychologically and physically for years beyond the end of their caregiving days, it is vitally important for care partners to be proactive in keeping stress levels as low as possible. The Alzheimer's Association provides valuable resources toward this end, as do organizations such as the National Alliance for Caregiving and the Family Caregiving Alliance.

Can care partners maintain self-esteem and avoid feelings of failure?

I have emphasized how important it is for people diagnosed with AD or other types of dementia to maintain feelings of self-worth and of self-esteem. This is no less true for healthy care partners, and it can be quite challenging for them to do so. When they are not well educated about the remaining cognitive and social strengths of their diagnosed loved ones, they often experience feelings of failure because, for example, they do not understand how to communicate effectively, how to use their loved one's abilities to the fullest degree, and how to avoid playing into their loved one's "weak suits." One spousal care partner, Mrs. U, expressed this feeling clearly, remarking about her husband diagnosed with dementia (Sabat, 2011):

> It saddens me to realize how little I know about helping (husband's name). ... A friend described me this way: I was like a fly looking for a way out and each time I hit a window and it was closed, I would try another and then another one. I told her that I have run out of windows. (p. 85)

Indeed, care partners often think that because they cannot make things all better, they cannot make things better at all. This idea is patently false. It is also one of the most important hurdles of misunderstanding that a healthy care partner must traverse.

My father was a deeply devoted care partner for my mother, Edythe, who was diagnosed with a vascular dementia. During one of my extended visits with them, he said to me, "I just want the old Edye back." It was clear, however, that she was never going to return completely to the way she was before small strokes damaged her brain to the degree that she was diagnosed with dementia. And so I had to tell him that even though that was not possible, he still could work with her remaining abilities so that the two of them could do their best under the circumstances. This was a way for him to understand that he still had the ability to help her to be as good as she could be and that that would help him too. Thus, he would say to her, "I need you to help me so that I can help you." Frequently, that was exactly the right thing to say. It can be very helpful, therefore, for healthy care partners to obtain counseling, which has been shown to aid in delaying placement of the person diagnosed into long-term care (Mittleman et al., 1996). As well, counseling and education have been found to reduce some of the stress and other negative effects of caregiving (Patterson & Grant, 2003; Quayhagen et al., 2000; Whitlatch et al., 2006). What care partners can learn about their loved ones and themselves can help to forestall the decision to place a loved one into long-term care.

Are there positive aspects to being a care partner?

Due to the tremendous focus on the profound stresses and strains of being a care partner to a person with dementia, the potentially positive aspects had been ignored for a long time (Kramer, 1997). Through education and counseling, some spousal care partners have discovered very positive aspects of themselves and also become aware more than ever before of the depth of their love for their spouse.

This was true for Mrs. U (Sabat, 2011), who was approximately 80 years old when her husband was diagnosed with dementia. Through education and counseling, she realized that she was not helping her husband as much as she wished:

> At times he resents my taking over his life completely and I resent having to do it. He also has physical problems and I am constantly worrying about his falling so I won't let him do anything (even taking out the garbage). . . . I thought that yelling would make him understand. (p. 85)

In this regard, she learned that it was extremely important to understand her husband's point of view: His life as an adult was all about being in command (he was a retired brigadier general), and because of the brain damage that led to his diagnosis, he was no longer in command of many aspects of his life. From his point of view, that was a huge, bitter pill to swallow. I explained to Mrs. U that his pride was injured and he likely needed to help out around the house—even taking out the garbage if nothing else—and that he had to have a sense of purpose given the person he had always been. Under the circumstances wherein she was taking over everything, it was easy for him to feel burdensome, and that was anathema to him. It was clear that he needed reassurance, for he said to her, "I know you never thought our life would come to this" (p. 85).

When Mrs. U understood her husband's point of view, she was able to treat him as she would wish to be treated if the situation were reversed. She commented,

> Treating (husband's name) with dignity is my goal. This morning he said, "Let me dress myself so I won't be a burden to you." He even washed some dishes for me standing at the sink. He also helped me with the taxes. I just can't find enough jobs for him. Also, he is returning his own phone calls. I was doing it before. (p. 88)

As a result of her new understanding and improved interactions with her husband, her adult children found her to be much calmer than she was on their previous visits. Her realization and acceptance of the fact that she could not fix everything was also extremely helpful especially given her personality for most of her adult life: "I am the type of person who likes to fix things, but I want to fix it and then move on to the next thing that needs to be fixed. And, of course, I can never fix (husband's name)" (p. 90). She came to understand that even though she could not make her husband all better, she could still help to make good moments happen for the two of them. She also worked at not resenting the fact that her husband was diagnosed with dementia. As she said, "Though there are . . .

times I do still resent what has happened to (husband's name), they are less frequent, and on some days I can almost believe there is a reason" (p. 90). She continued,

> You also explained to me that he was pushing me away and in turn was being angry with himself for being mean to me. He also was sad about the burden he was inflicting on me. All that you said eased my resentment toward him. ... You were accurate when you told me that the more I understood his point of view and the better I understood his condition, the less anxious I would feel and the more empathetic I would feel. (p. 91)

When Gen. U entered a nursing home, Mrs. U visited him every day and, in the process, became involved with other residents, bringing them good cheer and engaging them in a very respectful and energetic way. This led to her saying,

> I also feel I have a mission to make a difference in the nursing home, no matter how small. ... Just a smile and a kind word are so meaningful to most of the residents ... what is so neat about all this is that I can use these tools not only with (husband's name) but with others I encounter. (p. 92)

Thus, in the process of helping her husband, she found a way to be helpful to other nursing home residents, and this had a profoundly positive impact on her:

> It is like I found another person inside of me. I like the person I found. I am so happy with me most of the time. It takes so little to bring me joy and a smile to my face. Just having (one of the residents) smile at me and knowing that he is experiencing a little emotion, having (name of

another resident) talk to me and the others who respond
to my interest in them is like food for my soul. (p. 92)

She went on to say,

I get so much pleasure from doing what I can for the residents. . . . I sewed another button on BP's shirt and you
would think I had given him the best gift. He couldn't
stop thanking me and was so sorry he couldn't do anything for me. What he doesn't realize is that he *is* doing
something for me . . . you do know the good feeling you
get when you make someone happy. In this crazy world,
what could be better than that? (p. 92)

Simultaneously, Mrs. U experienced something of a revela-
tion regarding her relationship with her husband:

I have always known that he loved me even though he
very seldom expressed it, and I knew his career came
first. What I didn't know is how much I love him and
what I am willing to do for him and this experience is
revealing this to me. I am going to have to give this reve-
lation a lot of thought. (p. 93)

Thus, in the process of being a devoted care partner to her
husband while he was still living at home, Mrs. U learned more
about his condition, improved her ability to help him, felt less
stress, and found new, positive aspects of herself in the process.
After he entered a nursing home, she had more positive experiences by helping other residents, seeing and working with their
strengths, and bringing them good cheer. In so doing, she found
new aspects of herself that she liked very much. She found that
giving to others resulted in her feeling good as well, and she
and her husband also made good, sweet moments together that
were especially, mutually, gratifying. Working in positive ways

to help her husband and other residents enhanced her sense of control over the situations she faced as well as her feelings of self-worth as she applied the "Golden Rule." For Mrs. U, the experience of being a spousal care partner became one of ongoing growth that continued even after her husband died. She began attending weekly worship services, which was something she never did during her many decades of married life even though her husband always attended weekly services. She even joked about how he must be laughing at her taking the same seat he used every week during services. Perhaps, given her personality, it was not surprising that she found a place for spirituality in her life, but the question remains whether there is a place for spirituality in the lives of people with dementia.

Is there a place for spirituality in the lives of people with dementia?

Considering the variety and depth of the challenges that AD and other forms of dementia pose, it is hardly surprising that people diagnosed may feel angry, resentful, misunderstood, demeaned, stigmatized, patronized, and cheated out of years of their lives. They may question the faith with which they lived most of their lives, and they may even wonder what they did to deserve such a fate. The reactions people have are as varied as the personalities and lives of the people themselves.

Lisa Snyder (2003) explored the statements of 19 men and 9 women, 18 of whom were diagnosed with AD and 1 with frontotemporal dementia, concerning the place of spirituality in their lives. The group included 11 Protestants, 7 Catholics, 3 Christians of unnamed denomination, 3 Jews, and 3 Buddhists. Some statements came from interviews she conducted with people diagnosed, and others were collected and documented by other clinicians. She found general themes into which the statements could be grouped: finding meaning in AD, coping with AD, the effect of the disease on faith, and its effect on spiritual or religious practice.

Snyder (2003) found that there was no one faith or religious perspective that offered more to people in terms of their ability to find meaning in or cope with their illness. Indeed, there was no evidence that those with a religious or spiritual perspective coped better with dementia than did those who did not have a religious or faith-based practice in their lives. Some indicated that even though they were no longer able to participate in worship services due to memory dysfunction and/or motor dysfunction, their sense of the spiritual dimension in life had deepened. One man indicated that religion was not what he needed to get through AD; rather, it was the beauty and mystery of nature in the mountains and sunsets that was his "religion." Where some questioned, "Why me?" others did not. Where some wondered what kind of God would allow AD to exist, others did not. Where some were disillusioned because God did not answer their supplications for recovery, others were strengthened in their sense of gratitude to God for their good days and their families and prayed for the strength to endure the difficulties they faced, believing that God would never forsake them.

Other researchers have found that among people diagnosed with AD in the early stages according to standard tests, their lifelong faith and spiritual practices continued despite their diagnoses; they gave their days to their church, their faith, and the support of their families (Beuscher & Grando, 2009); and they believed that concentrating on the present, living with hope day by day, rather than on the future was also important (Stuckey et al., 2002). This could be accomplished, as some people believed, by slowing down so as to enjoy life more than in the past, as AD forced that slowing down to occur according to God's plan (Phinney et al., 2002; Stuckey et al., 2002).

The varied ways in which people cope with and understand their illness and its relation to their spiritual life or lack thereof encourage us to appreciate yet again the value of person-centered care so as to honor the points of view and needs of individuals and provide them with supportive care, nonjudgmental understanding, and non-anxious presence. There are organizations that provide for the pastoral and spiritual care for older people. One such organization, Meaningful Ageing Australia (http://meaningfulageing.org.au), formerly known as PASCOP (Pastoral and Spiritual Care of Older People), is dedicated to providing quality pastoral and spiritual care in all care settings by working with faith-based and non-faith-based organizations be they of the charitable or private-sector variety.

That people continue to think about the meaning of their illness and of their lives—and how to cope best with their situations—in spiritual, nonspiritual, or religiously oriented ways sheds light on what dementia does and does not entail. To put it concretely, a person may be unable to recall what she had for breakfast or her granddaughter's name, may be unable to do simple arithmetic or dress herself, and may still be able to discuss her relationship (or lack thereof) to God, what dementia means to her, and how she is going about coping with its effects. This should give us pause and encourage us to consider further what dementia *does not mean.*

7

AND IN THE END . . .

When one of our loved ones or someone whom we are trying to help professionally is diagnosed with Alzheimer's disease (AD) or another type of dementia, we are presented with what is often considered a terrible fate that ends with death. We can, however, look at this situation rather differently, just as we can look at life itself as being something other than the death sentence that it is, in fact. Although dementia may frighten us due to the decline it represents, we are all living with the certitude of death from the moment of our birth, and the process of decline will be ours whether or not we are diagnosed with dementia if we live long enough! Just the same, we need not live our days with the dread of decline and death dominating our thoughts. We can choose instead to live our lives with joy and a sense of adventure and gratitude, especially because each day may be our final day.

We can view the diagnosis as being a great challenge as well as an opportunity for us and for our loved ones. That is, we can decide to respond to this situation by working diligently and taking the time to identify each and every way that the person diagnosed is, indeed, a person who has important strengths and admirable attributes. We can communicate our desire and intention to help and to be with him or her in the most respectful, compassionate, humane way possible so as to ease that person's despair and fear as much as possible. We can act to provide him or her with feelings of safety and acceptance, to make good moments together, to share laughter as well as tears. We can act to tap into and respect the diagnosed person's strengths. The road to realizing these rather ambitious goals begins with keeping in the forefront of our minds the answers to the important question of what strengths can be retained by people with AD or another dementia.

What strengths can people with Alzheimer's disease or another dementia retain?

People diagnosed retain many of the strengths and abilities they enjoyed earlier in their lives. For example, they

- can make new memories even if the memories cannot be recalled in detail (as discussed previously, remembering is more than recalling; implicit memory can still work.);
- are sensitive to the emotions and vulnerability of others;
- can be embarrassed and humiliated;
- can work to maintain self-respect and dignity;
- can feel and show love for and gratitude toward others;
- can appreciate and yearn for the love and acceptance of others;
- wish not to be a burden to loved ones;
- need reassurance and compassion;
- can display and appreciate humor and other valued emotions;
- can evaluate social situations accurately;
- can feel loneliness and despair;
- can have spiritual experiences and retain religious perspectives;
- can have meaningful thoughts even if they are unexpressed in words;
- need to be appreciated for their virtues and forgiven for their foibles;
- are hurt by being ignored or treated as nonentities;

- can act out of intention and in meaningful ways in social situations;
- can make adaptations to compensate for problems due to brain damage;
- can recognize and remember the good intentions of others who try to understand, try to communicate, and show kindness;
- can communicate best when not anxious and when assured that interlocutors are listening;
- need to be able to act independently and to have choices;
- are aided by nonjudgmental people and the non-anxious presence of others;
- need to have purpose;
- need to be listened to and heard;
- retain selfhood in a variety of ways;
- can communicate via words as well as via actions if words fail;
- can express themselves creatively via art, music, and dance and benefit from doing so; and
- can experience fulfillment.

Almost all of these can be true of people who are not diagnosed, including healthy care partners. It may be quite accurate, then, to suggest that people diagnosed have more in common with healthy others than they have differences. How they express these points of commonality may vary, but the commonalities still exist. At the same time, however, there are those stark, disturbing differences, the dysfunctions, that lead to the diagnosis of dementia and that are strikingly recognizable to one or another degree.

How can we deal with those differences in ways that are effective for all concerned?

When a loved one, especially perhaps a parent or spouse, shows signs of physical and mental weakness, of dysfunction, it can be threatening, upsetting, and frightening, particularly if that person has always been an anchor for us—someone whose love and support have been ever present in our lives. And so when that loved one asks the same questions repeatedly after they have been answered already, wants to send a gift to a deceased parent, folds towels incorrectly and puts them "away" where they do not belong, leaves the stove burners on when they should be turned off, or is found standing naked in the kitchen in the middle of a cold winter night, we can feel terribly upset and simultaneously out of control because we feel powerless to make those problems go away and want desperately for all this not to be happening to someone whom we love. Or, perhaps, all this is happening to a parent or spouse with whom we have had a stormy relationship, and that surely can make matters tremendously difficult in still other ways. All these feelings may be accompanied by the thought that "this is not fair" to anyone, and we want to scream out in sad, threatened, frustrated agony. We want it all to stop. Unfortunately, all too frequently, we scream at the people diagnosed—because we do not want this for them or for ourselves, and if only they would stop repeating the same questions, if they would only answer us correctly when we ask, "What did you have for breakfast?" maybe we would all feel better—but the screaming serves only to make things worse for everyone. Cursing the darkness will not bring light to this situation.

Instead, it is critical first to remember the previously discussed strengths and decide to work at making the best of our lives together. This is the first step in taking control. Care partners' experiences can be affected by the degree to which they feel in control of situations. Research on locus of control (LoC) (Lachman, 1986; Shewchuk, Foelker, & Niederehe, 1990) illuminates the differences between internal and external LoC, with the former being one's belief that he or she controls situations more than does the external environment; external LoC is the opposite. Diminished internal LoC, related to learned helplessness (Seligman, 1975), has been linked to decreases in physical and mental health and higher mortality rates (Adamson & Shamale, 1965; Lieberman & Tobin, 1983; Schulz, 1976). Caregivers' feelings of burden may be connected partially to their own, and the care recipients', diminished internal LoC (Scholl & Sabat, 2008). That is, the feeling of being more burdened (and burdensome) can be increased if one feels increasingly out of control of situations. Feelings of self-worth can be affected by perceived success and failure in caregiving, and these can be linked in part to the caregiver's internal LoC. So the more we believe that we can control situations, the greater is our internal LoC, the greater is our sense of self-worth, and we experience failure less often. Of course, caring for a loved one with dementia can often inspire us to feel that there is very little we can control.

So how do we increase our internal locus of control?

We can begin by working diligently on the following:

1. Accepting the dementia-related deficits and not making them the most important aspects of our focus
2. Focusing instead on and then using the diagnosed person's remaining strengths
3. Seeing with great compassion the vulnerable person inside, remembering the love we feel and how that person is trying tenaciously to cope with the effects of brain damage that he or she never wanted in the first place
4. Remembering that the person diagnosed may have deeply injured pride and feel terribly embarrassed, even ashamed, and therefore in need of support

So we answer the repeated question each time as if it were the first time and remain calm and, perhaps, after having done that half a dozen times, reply by saying, "Take a guess" and perhaps he or she will guess correctly because implicit memory systems still work. Or, refold the towels and put them where they do belong, knowing that by letting him or her fold the towels, you did a good thing in giving your loved one a sense of purpose by doing something to be of help. Or, you can fold the towels together and ask your loved one to join you in putting the towels in their proper place—in multiple stages so that you are making the trip to that same closet a few times so as to reinforce the proper location. Or, if he or she insists that the small package on the table needs to be put in the refrigerator, put it in the refrigerator and remove it later if it really does not belong there. There is no need to get into a difficult discussion (that leads nowhere) about why the package does not belong in the refrigerator or that the towels are not folded correctly or that they do not belong in the bedroom closet. Your loved one is just trying to be helpful, wanting not to be a burden, and is doing the best that he or she can do, so allow that to happen and say "thanks" sincerely and lovingly. At the heart of all this is acceptance of the deficits that exist coupled with the desire to rise to the challenge and make things work to the best of one's ability with the calmest kindness and compassion one can muster. Everyone's blood pressure can thereby remain at healthy levels.

Is this easy to do?

No; surely not at the beginning. With diligent practice, focused attention, love, and compassion, however, it can become increasingly easier with time. In the end, if we are successful in at least some respects, whenever we look back at this time we will be glad that we made the effort to take this approach because we succeeded in making some good moments, and that is a legacy we will be proud to have created.

But what is really at the foundation of doing all this work?

One way to answer this question is found in an encounter I had after a presentation I gave as part of a caregivers education series at the Holy Cross Hospital Medical Adult Day Center in Silver Spring, Maryland. I spoke about the abilities that remain intact in people with AD, and at the end of my remarks, a young couple approached me, telling me that their parent (and in-law) who was diagnosed with probable AD was now living with them. They then asked me, "So you're saying that we shouldn't give up on people?" "Exactly correct," I answered. Everything else proceeds from this point of view, this belief: We must not give up on someone because of the deficits that exist due to brain damage caused by disease.

Why shouldn't we give up on people with Alzheimer's disease or another type of dementia?

One way to answer this question is to think of what inspired the question posed by the previously mentioned young couple and return to the list of strengths retained by people diagnosed. Given so many strengths, it would make just as little sense to give up on someone diagnosed as it would to give up on someone deemed healthy who possessed the same strengths. The fact that a person cannot recall the day of the week or asks the same question repeatedly, cannot recognize a relative by sight, calls her daughter "my mother" (due to word-finding problems), or says that the salami sandwich she just ate was the first time she had eaten one (even though her family had a deli market when she grew up and ate salami sandwiches all the time) does not mean that those previously listed strengths are gone, and it surely does not mean that the person has no self or that there is "no one home," as it were. People with AD or another type of dementia are still people, even though some aspects of their cognitive/ thinking ability have been damaged. Another example may be instructive.

A man had been diagnosed with frontotemporal lobar dementia, and one of the dysfunctions resulting from this kind of brain damage is primary progressive aphasia (PPA). In PPA, language abilities become slowly but increasingly impaired so that eventually the ability to speak is lost almost completely along with the ability to read, write, and understand spoken words. While he was being assessed by a speech pathologist, the man said, with tremendous effort, "P-P-A" and then made a "thumbs down" gesture. This situation was presented to me by that same speech pathologist during a question-and-answer period at a conference symposium, and he then asked me, "So what do I say to that?" I replied that if I were in that same situation, I would say something like,

> Yes, PPA really stinks (I used a different, nastier word) and if I could make it go away for you, I would do it instantly. I'm really sorry that I cannot do that, but I will work with you so that we can deal with this together as best we can.

The questioner thanked me and said, "That's a really good response." He shared my belief that the man who was diagnosed was still "there" and deserved to be commiserated with, validated, and treated with compassion. After all, the man made a very astute observation about his condition. Yes, he could not utter the words that would capture his feeling about his diagnosis and its meaning, but instead he used a gesture that captured his feeling perfectly. The inability to speak the correct words or to pronounce words correctly or to speak many words at all does not mean that the person involved has vanished.

When my mother was in her late 80s and diagnosed with a vascular dementia, she was confined to a wheelchair. She rarely spoke, but when I sat quietly with her, holding her hand, she often broke the silence by saying, "Please don't ever leave me." Words cannot capture the feeling of poignancy I experienced in those moments. I felt the same way when I had to put an adult diaper on her and saw the look on her face indicating that that was the last thing she'd ever wish for me to have to do for her. She was utterly vulnerable in so many ways and felt it keenly. Loving reassurance was what she needed and what I gave her. She was, after all, my mother.

There is much more to each of us than the losses of particular types of thinking ability involved in the diagnosis of dementia. As noted among the strengths listed previously, people diagnosed can experience fulfillment, but none of us can have that experience, even for a moment, without the solicitude of others.

John Killick provided a wonderful example in a letter he wrote to me about a woman diagnosed with dementia who lived in a nursing home:

> One day in my role of a poet I went to a care home to work with the residents. I was introduced to "Peachey," who talked very fluently and intensely about her life. I made a poem from her story, entirely in her own words. The following week I took the poem back to her, read it to her and gave her a copy. She immediately went round the home collecting the staff who were on duty. She arranged chairs in rows in a corridor, climbed on one herself, and whilst I held her, read the poem to them as if she were giving a performance in a theatre. Everyone clapped.
>
> The following week I returned to the home, and knocked on the door of her room. When I entered I saw that the staff had framed her poem and hung it on the wall. She pointed to it; "Read that!" she said. I walked over and was reading it to myself. "No, out loud!" she ordered. I read the poem. "What do you think of it?" she asked. "Brilliant" I answered. "I think so too" she said. "A kind man came here one day and wrote it down." She had no idea it was me!

PEACHEY

When we got off the plane
the man in the little hut
was selling the photographs he took.
He said "This is the lady."
He didn't need any building up of acquaintance.
It was straight from the horse's mouth.

I wasn't brill at school,
but the boys called after me ...
the boys christened me "Peachey."
And I didn't like it.
I didn't know it was a gift.
But the teacher had a soft spot;
he never said anything, of course,
but it was in his eyes.

I roar with laughing at people,
and they laugh at me.
But I don't know any jokes.
It's all home-made humour.
If it fits I say the phrase.
Sparsmodic. I can laugh and like it.

I used to sing for the people,
sing what fits the emotion at the time.
When I first did it
I thought I was going to be reprimanded
for singing out of line.
But Life is Singing.

I'll talk, but it's not my scene,
chatting somebody up.
I'm not a grabber of situations,
I come out in little phrases, that's me.
And I don't know anybody who's not cheerful.
I bet you've never been so near Nature before!

Peachey made a memory of a kind man who came to her room and wrote down her words now framed and displayed on the wall, but she did not recall that that man was John Killick, who was standing before her once again. John and Peachey made lovely moments together that each remembered in his and her own way; they provided a special kind of fulfillment for and with one another. Peachey found fulfillment in being appreciated, for being seen in ways that supported her feeling of proper pride, knowing that she could tell her life story and have it heard by an eager listener. It means so much to elders, regardless of diagnostic status, to be heard and appreciated as they think about and tell the story of their lives. John Killick found fulfillment in being able to use his sensitivity and talent as a writer, a poet, and a person who delights in helping people with dementia, such as Peachey, so that they can be heard; so that they can experience good moments; so that they can laugh, feel delight and warmth; and so that they can be themselves to the fullest extent possible and experience truly priceless renewals of the spirit.

How we understand and care for people diagnosed with AD or another type of dementia is related intimately to how we view them—"we" meaning family members, friends, and professional care providers. Many among our ranks today, however, could very well be among "those diagnosed" tomorrow.

A society can be judged by how it treats its most vulnerable members; people with dementia and their care partners are surely among them. John Killick listened to Peachey and to others and made their words into poems, Penny Harris organized an intergenerational choir, Elizabeth Lokon created the Opening Minds through Art program, Lisa Snyder listened to Bill and worked with others to create a support group for people diagnosed with AD, and Tena Alonzo helped change the culture of care at the Beatitudes Campus. Each of these is an admirable effort that does great good.

Should these efforts and others like them be expanded to a much larger scale so as to help the millions of people diagnosed and their care partners who could benefit greatly from such programs?

What sorts of private and local community, state, and federal government actions are needed to do so and thereby improve the quality of those millions of lives, and how can our political will be summoned toward that end?

What does the present less than optimal treatment of people with AD and other types of dementia say about us as human beings and the priorities of our society as a whole?

How do we—each of us—wish to be valued and treated?

What will our answers to the previous questions teach our children and grandchildren, who may one day be caring for us and for others?

Our answers to these and related questions will be reflected not only in our own quality of life but also in that of generations of others. We, therefore, have every reason to use the challenge presented by Alzheimer's Disease and other dementias as an opportunity to become the most humane human beings we can be. Hillel's words (*Ethics of the Fathers* 1:14) are apt: "If not now, when?"

REFERENCES

Adams, T. (2003). Developing an inclusive approach to dementia care. *Practice, 15,* 45–56.

Adams, T., & Gardiner, P. (2005). Communication and interaction within dementia care triads. *Dementia, 4,* 185–205.

Adamson, J., & Shamale, A. (1965). Object loss, giving up, and the onset of psychiatric disease. *Psychosomatic Medicine, 27,* 557–576.

Adolphs, R. (2005). What is special about social cognition? In J. T. Cacioppo (Ed.), *Social neuroscience: People thinking about people* (pp. 269–286). Boston, MA: MIT Press.

Albert, N. S., Naeser, M. A., Levine, H. L., & Garvey, J. (1984). Ventricular size in patients with dementia of the Alzheimer's type. *Archives of Neurology, 41,* 1258–1263.

Allan, K., & Killick, J. (2000). Undiminished possibility: The arts in dementia care. *Journal of Dementia Care, 8,* 16–18.

Allan, K., & Killick, J. (2014). Communication and relationships: An inclusive social world. In M. Downs & B. Bowers (Eds.), *Excellence in dementia care: Research into practice* (2nd ed., pp. 240–255). New York: McGraw-Hill.

American Psychiatric Association. (2013). *Diagnostic and statistical manual of mental disorders* (5th ed.). Arlington, VA: American Psychiatric Publishing.

Ballard, C., & Hulford, L. (2006). Drugs used to relieve the behavioral symptoms of dementia. In J. C. Hughes (Ed.), *Palliative care in severe dementia* (pp. 65–75). London, England: Quay Books.

Barber, S. J., Mather, M., & Gatz, M. (2015). How stereotype threat affects healthy older adults' performance on clinical assessments of cognitive decline: The key role of regulatory fit. *Journals of Gerontology: Psychological Sciences, 70,* 891–900.

Barr, R., & Hayne, H. (2000). Age-related changes in imitation: Implications for memory development. In C. Rovee-Collier, L. P. Lipsitt, & H. Hayne (Eds.), *Progress in infancy research* (Vol. 1, pp. 21–67). Mahwah, NJ: Erlbaum.

Basting, A. D. (2003). Exploring the creative potential of people with Alzheimer's disease and related dementia: Dare to imagine. In J. L. Ronch & J. G. Goldfield (Eds.), *Mental wellness in aging: Strengths-based approaches* (pp. 353–367). Baltimore, MD: Health Professions Press.

Basting, A. D. (2006). Arts in dementia care: "This is not the end. It's the end of this chapter." *Generations, 30,* 16–20.

Basting, A. D., & Killick, J. (2003). *The arts and dementia care: A resource guide.* Brooklyn, NY: National Center for Creative Aging.

Baudic, S., Dalla Barba, G., Thibaudet, M. C., Smagghe, A., Remy, P., & Traykov, L. (2006). Executive function deficits in early Alzheimer's disease and their relations with episodic memory. *Archives of Clinical Neuropsychology, 21,* 15–21.

Benjamin, B. J. (1999). Validation: A communicative alternative. In L. Volicer & L. Bloom-Charette (Eds.), *Enhancing the quality of life in advanced dementia* (pp. 107–125). Philadelphia, PA: Brunner/Mazel.

Beuscher, L., & Grando, V. T. (2009). Using spirituality to cope with early stage Alzheimer's disease. *Western Journal of Nursing Research, 31,* 583–598.

Blessed, G., Tomlinson, B. E., & Roth, M. (1968). The association between quantitative measures of dementia and of senile change in the grey matter of elderly subjects. *British Journal of Psychiatry, 114,* 797–811.

Borrie, C. (2015). *The long hello: Memory, my mother, and me.* New York, NY: Simon & Schuster.

Boyle, P. A., Buchman, A. S., Wilson, R. S., Yu, L., Schneider, J. A., & Bennett, D. A. (2012). Effect of purpose in life on the relation between Alzheimer disease pathologic changes on cognitive function in advanced age. *Archives of General Psychiatry, 69,* 499–506.

Brooker, D. (2006). *Person-centred dementia care: Making services better.* London, England: Kingsley.

Brooker, D. (2012). Understanding dementia and the person behind the diagnostic label. *International Journal of Person Centered Medicine, 2*(1), 11–17.

Brooker, D., La Fontaine, J., De Vries, K., & Latham, I. (2013). The development of PIECE-dem: Focussing on the experience of care for people living with advanced dementia. *British Psychological Society Clinical Psychology Forum, 250,* 38–46.

Buber, M. (1937). *I and thou* (R. Gregor Smith, trans). Edinburgh, Scotland: Clark.

Cheston, R., & Bender, M. (1999). *Understanding dementia: The man with the worried eyes.* London, England: Kingsley.

Cohen, D., & Eisdorfer, C. (2002). *The loss of self: A family resource for the care of Alzheimer's disease and related disorders* (rev. ed.). New York: Norton.

Cohen-Mansfield, J. (2014). Understanding behaviour. In M. Downs & B. Bowers (Eds.), *Excellence in dementia care: Research into practice* (2nd ed., pp. 220–239). New York, NY: McGraw-Hill.

Cohen-Mansfield, J., & Marx, M. S. (1992). The social network of the agitated nursing home resident. *Research on Aging, 14,* 110–123.

Cooney, E. (2001, October). Death in slow motion. *Harper's Magazine,* pp. 43–58.

Cooney, E. (2004). *Death in slow motion: A memoir of a daughter, her mother, and the beast called Alzheimer's.* New York, NY: HarperCollins.

Csikszentmihalyi, M. (1990). *Flow: The psychology of optimal experience.* New York, NY: Harper & Row.

Davidson, A. (2006). *A curious kind of widow: Loving a man with advanced Alzheimer's.* McKinleyville, CA: Fithian Press.

Davies-Thompson, J., Pancaroglu, R., & Barton, J. (2014). Acquired prosopagnosia: Structural basis and processing impairments. *Frontiers in Bioscience, 6,* 159–174.

De Bleser, R., & Weisman, H. (1986). The communicative impact of non-fluent aphasia on the dialogue behavior of linguistically unimpaired partners. In F. Lowenthal & F. Vandamme (Eds.), *Pragmatics and education* (pp. 273–285). New York, NY: Plenum.

de Medeiros, K., Saunders, P. A., Doyle, P. J., Mosby, A., & Van Haitsma, K. (2011). Friendships among people with dementia in long-term care. *Dementia, 11,* 363–381.

Dennett, D. C. (1988). The intentional stance in theory and practice. In A. Whiten & R. W. Byrne (Eds.), *Machiavellian intelligence* (pp. 180–202). Oxford, England: Oxford University Press.

Dick, M. B., Kean, M. L., & Sands, D. (1989). Memory for internally generated words in Alzheimer's type dementia: Breakdown in encoding and semantic memory. *Brain and Cognition, 9,* 88–108.

Downs, M., & Bowers, B. (2014). *Excellence in dementia care: Research into practice* (2nd ed.). New York, NY: McGraw-Hill.

Doyle, P. J., & Rubinstein, R. L. (2013). Challenges to the implementation of a person-centered ideal within a dementia-specific long-term care context. In J. Ronch & A. Weiner (Eds.), *Models and pathways for person-centered elder care* (pp. 293–314). Baltimore, MD: Health Professions Press.

Edwards, C., McDonnell, C., & Merl, H. (2013). An evaluation of a therapeutic garden's influence on the quality of life of aged care residents with dementia. *Dementia, 12,* 494–510.

Elvish, R., Burrow, S., Cawley, R., Harney, K., Graham, P., Pilling, M., . . . Keady, J. (2014). Getting to know me: The development and evaluation of a training programme for enhancing skills in the care of people with dementia in general hospital settings. *Aging and Mental Health, 18,* 481–488.

Fleischman, D. A., Gabrieli, J. D. E., Rinaldi, J. A., Reminger, S. L., Grinnell, E. R., Lange, K. L., & Shapiro, R. (1997). Word-stem completion priming for perceptually and conceptually encoded words in patients with Alzheimer's disease. *Neuropsychologia, 35,* 25–35.

Franzen, J. (2001, September 10). My father's brain: What Alzheimer's takes away. *The New Yorker,* pp. 81–91.

Fritsch, T., Kwak, J., Grant, S., Lang, J., Montgomery, R. R., & Basting, A. (2009). Impact of TimeSlips, a creative expression intervention program, on nursing home residents with dementia and their caregivers. *The Gerontologist, 49,* 117–127.

Fuchs, E. (2005, May 8). Alzheimer's: A mother–daughter act. *The New York Times.*

Fukushima, T., Nagahata, K., Ishibashi, N., Takahashi, Y., & Moriyama, M. (2005). Quality of life from the viewpoint of patients with dementia in Japan: Nurturing through an acceptance of dementia by patients, their families and care professionals. *Health and Social Care in the Community, 13,* 30–37.

Gawande, A. (2014). *Being mortal: Medicine and what matters in the end.* New York, NY: Metropolitan Books.

Giannakopoulos, P., Hof, P. R., Giannakopoulos, A., Herrmann, F. R., Michel, J., & Bouras, C. (1995). Regional distribution of neurofibrillary tangles and senile plaques in the cerebral cortex of very old patients. *Archives of Neurology, 52,* 1150–1159.

Green, R. C., Goldstein, F. C., Mirra, S. S., Alazraki, N. P., Baxt, J. L., & Bakay, R. A. (1995). Slowly progressive apraxia in Alzheimer's disease. *Journal of Neurology, Neurosurgery, and Psychiatry, 59,* 312–315.

Grosse, D. A., Wilson, R. S., & Fox, J. H. (1990). Preserved word stem completion priming of semantically encoded information in Alzheimer's disease. *Psychology and Aging, 5,* 304–306.

Hamington, M. (2004). *Embodied care: Jane Addams, Maurice Merleau-Ponty, and feminist ethics.* Urbana, IL: University of Illinois Press.

Harré, R. (1983). *Personal being.* Oxford, England: Blackwell.

Harré, R. (1991). The discursive production of selves. *Theory and Psychology, 1,* 51–63.

Harris, P. B. (2004). The perspective of younger people with dementia: Still an overlooked population. *Social Work in Mental Health, 2,* 17–36.

Harris, P. B. (2012). Maintaining friendships in early stage dementia: Factors to consider. *Dementia, 11,* 305–314.

Harris, P. B. (2016). Resilience and living well with dementia. In C. Clarke & E. Wolverson (Eds.), *Positive psychology approaches to dementia* (pp. 133–151). London, England: Kingsley.

Harris, P. B., & Caporella, C. A. (2014). An intergenerational choir formed to lessen Alzheimer's disease stigma in college students and decrease the social isolation of people with Alzheimer's disease and their family members: A pilot study. *American Journal of Alzheimer's Disease and Other Dementias, 29,* 270–281.

Harris, P. B., & Keady, J. (2004). Living with early-onset dementia: Exploring the experience and developing evidence-based guidelines for practice. *Alzheimer's Care Quarterly, 5,* 111–122.

Hawthorne, G. (2006). Measuring social isolation in older adults: Development and initial validation of the friendship scale. *Social Indicators Research, 77,* 521–548.

Hayne, H., Boniface, J., & Barr, R. (2000). The development of declarative memory in human infants: Age-related changes in deferred imitation. *Behavioral Neuroscience, 114,* 77–83.

Hill, H. (2003). A space to be myself. *Signpost, 7*(3), 37–39.

Howard, D. V. (1991). Implicit memory: An expanding picture of cognitive aging. *Annual Review of Gerontology and Geriatrics, 11,* 1–22.

Hubbard, G., Cook, A., Tester, S., & Downs, M. (2002). Beyond words: Older people with dementia using and interpreting nonverbal behavior. *Journal of Aging Studies, 16,* 155–167.

Hughes, J. C. (2011). *Thinking through dementia.* Oxford, England: Oxford University Press.

Hughes, J. C. (2014). *How we think about dementia.* London, England: Kingsley.

Hughes, J. C., & Baldwin, C. (2006). *Ethical issues in dementia care: Making difficult decisions.* London, England: Kingsley.

Hughes, J. C., Louw, S. J., & Sabat, S. R. (Eds.). (2006). *Dementia: Mind, meaning, and the person.* Oxford, England: Oxford University Press.

Hurd, M. D., Martorell, P., Delavande, A., Mullen, K. J., & Langa, K. M. (2013). Monetary costs of dementia in the United States. *New England Journal of Medicine, 368,* 1326–1334.

Ice, G. H. (2002). Daily life in a nursing home: Has it changed in 25 years? *Journal of Aging Studies, 16,* 345–359.

Jones, E. E., & Harris, V. A. (1967). The attribution of attitudes. *Journal of Experimental Social Psychology, 3,* 1–24.

Kahn, R. (1971). *The boys of summer.* New York, NY: Harper & Row.

Kahn-Dennis, K. (2002). The person with dementia and artwork: Art therapy. In P. B. Harris (Ed.), *The person with Alzheimer's disease: Pathways to understanding the experience* (pp. 246–269). Baltimore, MD: Johns Hopkins University Press.

Keady, J., Jones, L., Ward, R., Koch, S., Swarbrick, C., Hellstrom, I., . . . Williams, S. (2012). Introducing the bio-psycho-social model of dementia through a collective case study design. *Journal of Clinical Nursing, 22,* 2768–2777.

Kiecolt-Glaser, J. K., Preacher, J. K., MacCallum, R. C., Atkinson, C., Malarkey, W. B., & Glaser, R. (2003). Chronic stress and age-related increases in the proinflammatory cytokine IL-6. *Proceedings of the National Academy of Sciences of the USA, 100,* 9090–9095.

Killick, J. (1997). *You are words.* London, England: Hawker.

Killick, J. (2000). *Openings: Dementia poems and photographs.* London, England: Hawker.

Killick, J. (2008). *Dementia diary: Poems and prose.* London, England: Hawker.

Killick, J. (2012). *Playfulness and dementia: A practical guide.* London, England: Kingsley.

Killick, J. (2016). Creativity and dementia. In C. Clarke & E. Wolverson (Eds.), *Positive psychology approaches to dementia* (pp. 175–195). London, England: Kingsley.

Kitwood, T. (1995). Positive long-term changes in dementia: Some preliminary observations. *Journal of Mental Health, 4,* 133–144.

Kitwood, T. (1998). *Dementia reconsidered: The person comes first.* Philadelphia, PA: Open University Press.

Knopman, D. S., Parisi, J. E., Salviati, A., Foriach-Robert, M., Boeve, B. F., Ivnik, R. J., . . . Petersen, R. C. (2003). Neuropathology of cognitively normal elderly. *Journal of Neuropathology and Experimental Neurology, 62,* 1087–1095.

Kontos, P. (2004). Ethnographic reflections on selfhood, embodiment and Alzheimer's disease. *Ageing and Society, 24,* 829–849.

Kontos, P. (2005). Embodied selfhood in Alzheimer's disease: Rethinking person-centred care. *Dementia, 4,* 553–570.

Kontos, P. C. (2012). Rethinking sociability in long-term care: An embodied dimension of selfhood. *Dementia, 11,* 329–346.

Kramer, B. (1997). Gain in the caregiving experience: Where are we? What's next? *The Gerontologist, 37,* 218–232.

Kutner, N. G., Brown, P. J., Stavisky, R. C., Clark, W. S., & Green, R. C. (2000). "Friendship" interactions and expression of agitation among residents of a dementia care unit: Six-month observational data. *Research on Aging, 22,* 188–205.

Lachman, M. E. (1986). Locus of control in aging research: A case for multidimensional and domain specific assessment. *Psychology and Aging, 1,* 34–40.

Langer, E. J., & Rodin, J. (1976). The effects of choice and enhanced personal responsibility for the aged: A field experiment in an institutional setting. *Journal of Personality and Social Psychology, 34,* 191–198.

Lavretsky, H. (2014). *Resilience and ageing research and practice.* Baltimore, MD: Johns Hopkins University Press.

Levy, B. (1996). Improving memory in old age through implicit self-stereotyping. *Journal of Personality and Social Psychology, 71,* 1092–1107.

Lieberman, M. A., & Tobin, S. S. (1983). *The experience of old age: Stress, coping, and survival.* New York, NY: Basic Books.

Lokon, E., & Dana, C. (2014, January–February). Using art to overcome cognitive barriers. *Leading Age Magazine, 4,* 1–6.

Lokon, E., Kinney, J. M., & Kunkel, S. (2012). Building bridges across age and cognitive barriers through art: College students' reflections on an intergenerational program with elders who have dementia. *Journal of Intergenerational Relationships, 10,* 337–354.

Maher, B. (1970). *Principles of psychopathology.* New York, NY: McGraw-Hill.

Mak, W. (2010). Self-reported goal pursuit and purpose in life among people with dementia. *Journals of Gerontology Series B: Psychological Sciences and Social Sciences, 66B,* 177–184.

Matthews, E., Farrell, G., & Blackmore, A. (1996). Effects of an environmental manipulation emphasizing client-centred care on agitation and sleep in dementia sufferers in a nursing home. *Journal of Advanced Nursing, 24,* 439–447.

McKhann, G. M., Knopman, D. S., Chertkow, H., Hyman, B. T., Jack, C. R., Jr., Kawas, C. H., . . . Phelps, C. W. (2011). The diagnosis of dementia due to Alzheimer's disease: Recommendations from the National Institute on Aging–Alzheimer's Association workgroup on diagnostic guidelines for Alzheimer's disease. *Alzheimer's and Dementia, 7,* 263–269.

Mead, R. (2013, May 20). The sense of an ending. *The New Yorker,* pp. 92–103.

Mittleman, M. S., Ferris, S. H., Shulman, E., & Steinberg, G. (1996). A family intervention to delay nursing home placement of patients with Alzheimer disease. *JAMA, 276,* 1725–1731.

Moore, J. (2016). What is the sense of agency and why does it matter? *Frontiers in Psychology, 7.* Retrieved from http://dx.doi.org/10.3389/fpsyg.2016.01272

Morris, R. G., & Kopelman, M. D. (1986). The memory deficits in Alzheimer's type dementia: A review. *Quarterly Journal of Experimental Psychology, 38A,* 575–602.

Moyle, W., Venturato, L., Cooke, M., Murfield, J., Griffiths, S., Hughes, J., & Wolf, N. (2016). Evaluating the capabilities model of dementia care: A non-randomized controlled trial exploring resident quality of life and care staff attitudes and experiences. *International Psychogeriatrics, 28,* 1091–1100.

National Institute on Aging. (2003, December). *Alzheimer's disease: Unraveling the mystery* (No. 02-3782). Bethesda, MD: National Institutes of Health.

Nolan, M. R., Davies, S., Brown, J., Keady, J., & Nolan, J. (2004). Beyond "person-centred care": A new vision gerontological nursing. *International Journal of Older People Nursing, 13,* 45–53.

Partridge, F. M., Knight, R. G., & Feehan, M. (1990). Direct and indirect memory performance in patients with senile dementia. *Psychological Medicine, 20,* 111–118.

Patterson, T. L., & Grant, I. (2003). Interventions for caregiving in dementia: Physical outcomes. *Current Opinion in Psychiatry, 16,* 629–633.

Perani, D., Bressi, S., Cappa, S. F., Vallar, G., Alberoni, M., Grassi, F., . . . Fazio, F. (1993). Evidence of multiple memory systems in the human brain. *Brain, 116,* 903–919.

Phinney, A., Wallhagen, M., & Sands, L. P. (2002). Exploring the meaning of symptom awareness and unawareness in dementia. *Journal of Neuroscience Nursing, 34,* 79–90.

Power, G. A. (2010). *Dementia beyond drugs.* Baltimore, MD: Health Professions Press.

Pringle, D. (2003). Discourse: Making moments matter. *Canadian Journal of Nursing Research, 35,* 7–13.

Quayhagen, M. P., Quayhagen, M., Corbeil, R. R., Hendrix, R. C., Jackson, J. E., Snyder, L., & Bower, D. (2000). Coping with dementia: Evaluation of four nonpharmacologic interventions. *International Psychogeriatrics, 12,* 249–265.

Raia, P. (1999). Habilitation therapy: A new starscape. In L. Volicer & L. Bloom-Charette (Eds.), *Enhancing the quality of life in advanced dementia* (pp. 21–37). Philadelphia, PA: Brunner/Mazel.

Randolph, C., Tierney, M. C., & Chase, T. N. (1995). Implicit memory in Alzheimer's disease. *Journal of Clinical and Experimental Neuropsychology, 17,* 343–351.

Richards, K., Sullivan, S., Phillips, R., Beck, C. K., & Overton-McCoy, A. L. (2001). Effect of individualized activities on the sleep of nursing home residents who are cognitively impaired elders: A pilot study. *Journal of Gerontological Nursing, 27,* 30–37.

Russo, R., & Spinnler, H. (1994). Implicit verbal memory in Alzheimer's disease. *Cortex, 30,* 359–375.

Rusted, J., Sheppard, L., & Waller, D. (2006). A multi-centre randomized control group trial on the use of art therapy for older people with dementia. *Group Analysis, 39,* 517–536.

Sabat, S. R. (1991). Facilitating conversation via indirect repair: A case study of Alzheimer's disease. *Georgetown Journal of Languages and Linguistics, 2,* 284–296.

Sabat, S. R. (2001). *The experience of Alzheimer's disease: Life through a tangled veil.* Oxford, England: Blackwell.

Sabat, S. R. (2003). Some potential benefits of creating research partnerships with people with Alzheimer's disease. *Research Policy and Planning, 21,* 5–12.

Sabat, S. R. (2006). Implicit memory and people with Alzheimer's disease: Implications for caregiving. *American Journal of Alzheimer's Disease and Other Dementias, 21,* 11–14.

Sabat, S. R. (2011). Flourishing of the self while caring for a person with dementia: A case study of education, counseling, and psychosocial support via email. *Dementia, 10,* 81–97.

Sabat, S. R., & Cagigas, X. E. (1997). Extralinguistic communication compensates for the loss of verbal fluency: A case study of Alzheimer's disease. *Language and Communication, 17,* 341–351.

Sabat, S. R., Fath, H., Moghaddam, F. M., & Harré, R. (1999). The maintenance of self-esteem: Lessons from the culture of Alzheimer's sufferers. *Culture and Psychology, 5,* 5–31.

Sabat, S. R., & Harré, R. (1992). The construction and deconstruction of self in Alzheimer's disease. *Ageing and Society, 12,* 443–461.

Sabat, S. R., & Harré, R. (1994). The Alzheimer's disease sufferer as a semiotic subject. *Philosophy, Psychiatry, Psychology, 1,* 145–160.

Sabat, S. R., & Lee, J. M. (2012). Relatedness among people diagnosed with dementia: Social cognition and the possibility of friendship. *Dementia, 11,* 311–323.

Sachweh, S. (2008). *Spurenlesen im Sprachdschungel: Kommunikation und Verständigung mit demenzkranken Menschen* [*Following trails in the language jungle: Understanding and communicating with people with dementia*]. Bern, Switzerland: Huber.

Sacks, O. (1985). *The man who mistook his wife for a hat and other clinical tales.* New York, NY: Summit Books.

Sauer, P. E., Fopma-Loy, J., Kinney, J. M., & Lokon, E. (2016). "It makes me feel like myself": Person-centered versus traditional visual arts activities for people with dementia. *Dementia, 15*(5), 895–912.

Saunders, P. A., de Medeiros, K., Doyle, P., & Mosby, A. (2011). The discourse of friendship: Mediators of communication among dementia residents in long-term care. *Dementia, 11,* 347–361.

Schacter, D. L. (1987). Implicit memory: History and current status. *Journal of Experimental Psychology: Learning, Memory, and Cognition, 13,* 501–518.

Scholl, J. M., & Sabat, S. R. (2008). Stereotypes, stereotype threat and ageing: Implications for the understanding and treatment of people with Alzheimer's disease. *Ageing and Society, 28,* 103–130.

Scholzel-Dorenbos, C. J. M., Ettema, T. P., Bos, J., Boelens-van der Knoop, E., Gerritsen, D. L., Hoogeveen, F., . . . Droes, R. M. (2007). Evaluating the outcome of interventions on quality of life in dementia: Selection of the appropriate scale. *International Journal of Geriatric Psychiatry, 22,* 511–519.

Schulz, R. (1976). Effects of control and predictability on the psychology of the institutionalized aged. *Journal of Personality and Social Psychology, 33,* 563–573.

Seligman, M. (1975). *Helplessness: On depression, development, and death.* San Francisco, CA: Freeman.

Semuels, A. (2015, April 21). Building better nursing homes. *The Atlantic.* Retrieved from https://www.theatlantic.com/business/archive/2015/04/a-better-nursing-home-exists/390936

Shewchuk, R. M., Foelker, G. A., & Niederehe, G. (1990). Measuring locus of control in elderly persons. *International Journal of Aging and Human Development, 30,* 213–224.

Slavin, M. J., Mattingly, J. B., Bradshaw, J. L., & Storey, E. (2002). Local–global processing in Alzheimer's disease: An examination of interference, inhibition, and priming. *Neuropsychologia, 40,* 1173–1186.

Smith, G. C., & Hayslip, B. (2012). Resilience in adulthood and later life. *Annual Review of Gerontology and Geriatrics: Emerging Perspectives on Resilience in Later Life, 32*(1), 1–28.

Snowden, D. (1997). Aging and Alzheimer's disease: Lessons from the nun study. *The Gerontologist, 37,* 150–156.

Snyder, L. (2001). The lived experience of Alzheimer's: Understanding the feelings and subjective accounts of persons with the disease. *Alzheimer's Care Quarterly, 2,* 8–22.

Snyder, L. (2003). Satisfactions and challenges in spiritual faith and practice for persons with dementia. *Dementia: The International Journal of Social Research and Practice, 2,* 299–313.

Snyder, L. (2009). *Speaking our minds: What it's like to have Alzheimer's* (rev. ed.). Baltimore, MD: Health Professions Press.

Snyder, L., Jenkins, C., & Joosten, L. (2007). Effectiveness of support groups for people with mild to moderate Alzheimer's disease: An evaluative survey. *American Journal of Alzheimer's Disease and Other Dementias, 22,* 14–19.

Spaan, P. E. J., Raaijmakers, J. G. W., & Jonker. C. (2003). Alzheimer's disease versus normal aging: A review of the efficiency of clinical and experimental memory measures. *Journal of Clinical and Experimental Neuropsychology, 25,* 216–233.

Squire, L. R. (1994). Declarative and nondeclarative memory: Multiple brain systems supporting learning and memory. In D. L. Schacter & E. Tulving (Eds.), *Memory systems* (pp. 203–232). Cambridge, MA: MIT Press.

Stam, F., Wigboldus, J., & Smeulders, A. (1986). Age incidence of senile brain amyloidosis. *Pathology, Research and Practice, 181,* 558–562.

Steele, C. M. (1997). A threat in the air: How stereotypes shape intellectual identity and performance. *American Psychologist, 52,* 613–629.

Sterin, G. J. (2002). Essay on a word: A lived experience of Alzheimer's disease. *Dementia, 1,* 7–10.

Stern, Y. (2012). Cognitive reserve in aging and Alzheimer's disease. *Lancet Neurology, 11,* 1006–1012.

Stuckey, J. C., Post, S. G., Ollerton, S., FallCreek, S. J., & Whitehouse, P. J. (2002). Alzheimer's disease, religion, and the ethics of respect for spirituality: A community dialogue. *Alzheimer's Care Quarterly, 3,* 199–207.

Swaffer, K. (2015). Dementia and prescribed disengagement. *Dementia, 14,* 3–6.

Tomlinson, B. E., Blessed, G., & Roth, M. (1968). Observations on the brains of non-demented old people. *Journal of Neurological Science, 7,* 331–336.

Tomlinson, B. E., Blessed, G., & Roth, M. (1970). Observations on the brains of demented old people. *Journal of Neurological Science, 11,* 205–242.

van der Spek, K., Gerritsen, D. L., Smalbrugge, M., Nelissen-Vrancken, M. H., Wetzels, R. B., Smeets, C. H., . . . Koopmans, R. T. (2016). Only 10% of psychotropic drug use for neuropsychiatric symptoms in patients with dementia is fully appropriate. The PROPER-I Study. *International Psychogeriatrics, 28,* 1589–1595.

Ward, R., Howorth, M., Wilkinson, H., Campbell, S., & Keady, J. (2011). Supporting the friendships of people with dementia. *Dementia, 11,* 287–303.

Washburn, A. M., Sands, L. P., & Walton, P. J. (2003). Assessment of social cognition in frail older adults and its association with social functioning in the nursing home. *The Gerontologist, 43,* 203–212.

Weaks, D., Johnson, R., Wilkinson, H., & McLeod, J. (2009). *Developing nursing practice: A counselling approach to delivering postdiagnostic dementia.* Edinburgh, Scotland: Burdett Trust for Nursing, NHS Tayside, and the Universities of Abertay Dundee and Edinburgh.

Whitehouse, P. J. (2008). *The myth of Alzheimer's disease: What you aren't being told about today's most dreaded diagnosis.* New York, NY: St. Martin's Press.

Whitlatch, C. J., Judge, K., Zarit, S. H., & Femia, E. (2006). Dyadic intervention for family caregivers and care receivers in early-stage dementia. *The Gerontologist, 46,* 688–694.

Windle, G. (2012). The contribution of resilience to health ageing. *Perspectives in Public Health, 132,* 159–160.

Wolverson, E., Clarke, C., & Moniz-Cook, E. (2010). Remaining hopeful in early-stage dementia: A qualitative study. *Aging and Mental Health, 14,* 450–460.

Wolverson, E., & Patterson, K. (2016). Growth. In C. Clarke & E. Wolverson (Eds.), *Positive psychology approaches to dementia* (pp.152–174). London, England: Kingsley.

World Health Organization. (2015). *Dementia fact sheet.* Retrieved from http://www.who.int/mediacentre/factsheets/fs362/en

Yamashita, T., Kinney, J. M., & Lokon, E. (2011). The impact of a gerontology course and a service-learning program on college students' attitudes toward people with dementia. *Journal of Applied Gerontology, 32,* 139–163.

Yee-Melichar, D. (2011). Resilience in ageing: Cultural and ethnic perspectives. In B. Resnick, L. P. Gwyther, & K. A. Roberto (Eds.), *Resilience in aging: Concepts, research and outcomes* (pp. 133–146). New York, NY: Springer.

Younger, D., & Martin, G. (2000). Dementia care mapping: An approach to quality audit of services for people with dementia in two health districts. *Journal of Advanced Nursing, 32,* 1206–1212.

Zarit, S. H., Kim, K., Femia, E. E., Almeida, D. M., & Klein, L. C. (2014). The effects of adult day services on family caregivers' daily stress, affect, and health: Outcomes from the Daily Stress and Health (DaSH) study. *The Gerontologist, 54*(4), 570–579.

Zhang, Y. B., Harwood, J., Williams, A., Ylanne-McEwen, V., Wadleigh, P. M., & Thimm, C. (2006). The portrayal of older adults in advertising: A cross-national review. *Journal of Language and Social Psychology, 25,* 264–282.

INDEX